# ACQUAINTED
# WITH
# THE
# NIGHT

## The Image of Journalists in American Fiction, 1890-1930

by

## HOWARD GOOD

The Scarecrow Press, Inc.
Metuchen, N.J., & London
1986

The author gratefully acknowledges permission to reprint the poem on page iii: From The Poetry of Robert Frost edited by Edward Connery Lathem. Copyright 1928, 1969 by Holt, Rinehart and Winston. Copyright © 1956 by Robert Frost. Reprinted by permission of Henry Holt and Company.

Library of Congress Cataloging-in-Publication Data

Good, Howard, 1951–
    Acquainted with the night.

    Bibliography: p.
    Includes index.
    1. American fiction--20th century--History and criticism. 2. Journalists in literature. 3. Journalism in literature. 4. Newspapers in literature. 4. Newspapers in literature. 5. American fiction--19th century--History and criticism. I. Title.
    PS374.J68G66   1986        813'.52 09352097        86-3829
    ISBN 0-8108-1889-2

I have been one acquainted with the night.
I have walked out in rain--and back in rain.
I have outwalked the furthest city light.

I have looked down the saddest city lane.
I have passed by the watchman on his beat
And dropped my eyes, unwilling to explain.

--Robert Frost

To Barbara

Sail on, silver bird

## ACKNOWLEDGMENTS

George Orwell once compared writing a book to a "long bout of some painful illness," and unfortunately, he was not exaggerating. I want to express my thanks to those who helped me pull through. Professor Marion Marzolf of the University of Michigan listened with patience and sympathy to my theories, problems, and doubts as I struggled to turn a thousand pages of notes into a dissertation and then a dissertation into a book. My parents, Lillie and Samuel Good, sustained me not only with generous "grants" but also with their love and understanding and the example of their own fortitude. My young sons, Gabriel and Graham, provided much-needed comic relief from the headaches of rewriting. My wife, Barbara, sacrificed her security and happiness to support my work. She tolerated me when I was preoccupied and calmed me when I was slamming doors and furniture in frustration. She showed me the whole glorious rainbow of her heart.

# CONTENTS

## PREFACE

The big clock on the wall said one in the morning. I was alone in the <u>Observer</u> newsroom. The others had gone home or had scattered to their favorite bars. But I had pulled the lobster trick again. I was supposed to monitor the wires for late-breaking stories and approve the front page before the final edition went to press.

Hunched over the keyboard of my VDT, I checked the queues. There was a momentary lull in the phantasmagoria of murders and riots and earthquakes and plane crashes. Every time I called up the directory of another wire, the same message flashed on the screen: queue empty ... empty ... empty. It seemed in the silent, deserted newsroom a haunting cry, a premonition of loss.

Not many months later, I quit journalism and went off to teach at a Midwestern university. I had entered newspaper work because I mistook it for a back door to literature. Since I was fifteen, I had wanted to be a writer. What quicker way to get to know the world, I thought, than as a reporter on a big-city daily.

I got to know the world, but from the swaybacked chair of a wire editor. I was, as a reporter acquaintance sneeringly put it, a "deskoid." Caught in an electronic maze of news budgets, advisories, subgrafs, and urgents, I had no time or opportunity to learn to write better; if anything, I learned to write worse. I am still trying to overcome the bizarre literary tics I developed from churning out headline after headline night after night.

Perhaps what I was really fleeing when I left journalism was myself. "Does the business kill its best men?" asked Stanley Walker, city editor of the New York Herald Tribune in the 1920s. Straightaway he answered, "Sometimes, but it is more likely that the test lies in the man, that each man carries his guillotine or his wreath of laurel in his own typewriter." I was afraid that one day I would look into the wastebasket by my desk and find my head lying inside.

Every book reflects the predilections and perplexities of its author, but some books do so more obviously than others. My study of newspaper fiction is, in a sense, a self-study. Like many of the characters in the novels and short stories, I was attracted to journalism by the promise of romance and experience. Like them, I toiled long and hard to master my craft. And like them, I lost my enthusiasm for the work after a few years and got out.

My goal in the following pages is not to defend or debunk the literary image of journalists but to explain, as cogently as I can, what I found in the fables of now-forgotten writers. I must believe that my time in journalism sensitized me to the undercurrents of emotion and meaning in newspaper fiction. Popular literature can tell us a lot--and much of it wrenching--about the relationship between the public and the press and about the inner lives of journalists. We have only to listen with an open mind to the faded voices speaking out of history and dreams.

ACQUAINTED WITH THE NIGHT

## Chapter I

## INTRODUCTION

A devious affair, journalism.  But interesting!
--Floyd Dell, Moon-Calf

"A reporter is no hero for a novel," Stephen Crane scrawled in exasperation on a postcard as he struggled to complete Active Service (1899), his novel with a reporter for its hero.[1] Crane may have been right.  At least the journalist is portrayed in highly ambivalent terms in American fiction published from 1890 to 1930.  He was created in the imperfect image of his controversial profession.

The emergence of newspaper fiction in the 1890s as a distinct genre followed the emergence of the reporter as a distinct type.  "Social changes," George Santayana once said, "do not reach artistic expression until after their momentum is acquired and their other collateral effects are fully predetermined."[2]  In the last quarter of the nineteenth century, American journalism rapidly gathered momentum.  The newspaper was becoming a mass medium.  Yellow journals reached out with shorter, livelier stories, bigger, blacker headlines, and more pictures to a newly discovered audience of errand boys, factory girls, and raw immigrants.  Between 1870 and 1890, the total circulation of daily newspapers in the United States rose 222 percent, while the total population of the country rose only 63 percent.[3]

"There is no substitute for circulation," declared William Randolph Hearst, publisher of a string of yellow journals.[4]

Huge circulations were needed to defray soaring production costs. "The magnitude of the financial operations of the newspaper," Lincoln Steffens wrote in 1897, "is turning journalism upside down."[5] The age of personal journalism, of the editor-publisher who stamped his idiosyncrasies and beliefs on every facet of his newspaper, was ending as the press grew increasingly complex and commercial. By 1910, Edward Alsworth Ross was complaining in Atlantic Monthly, "More and more the owner of the big daily is a business man who finds it hard to see why he should run his property on different lines from the hotel proprietor, the vaudeville manager, or the owner of an amusement park. The editors are hired men, and they put into the paper no more of their conscience and ideals than comports with getting the biggest return from the investment."[6] And that could be big indeed. Advertising revenue climbed from about $90 million a year in 1890 to more than $600 million in 1920.[7]

When the press began to turn from a select readership of businessmen and professionals to a mass readership of factory workers and immigrants, the role of reporters expanded. For the first time, they were "actors in the drama of the newspaper world."[8] Metropolitan dailies relied on large numbers of them to gather and write stories of sex, violence, scandal, tragedy, and farce. Their new prominence was reflected in the growing use of bylines, which were frequent by 1886 in the New York World, the Boston Globe, and several other papers.[9] As Ned Brown, who abandoned medical studies to become a sports reporter for the World, recalled: "Being a newspaper writer gave you stature then, everywhere except in society. But elsewhere, a first-string reporter of any recognized paper ... had a lot of prestige.... He was a citizen of no mean state."[10]

Although newspaper owners were coming to view journalism as simply a moneymaking proposition, reporters and editors were coming to view it as something of a profession. In 1903, Julian Ralph, one of the leading reporters of his day, noted that journalism was once "a haphazard, unmethodical business, managed by printers and led by geniuses, ne'er-do-wells, Bohemians--often men of disorderly lives or irresponsible natures." Now, he added, "all newspaper men must be ready to work at every moment of every day; they must be sober; they must appear well, and they must be able at least to present the external signs of refinement."[11]

Besides being better mannered and better dressed than their predecessors, they were usually better educated. "It was not very many years ago," the trade magazine Journalist said in 1900, "that Horace Greeley made a remark to the effect that he would rather have a wild bull in his office than a college graduate. Today college bred men are the rule."[12] The Wharton School of Business at the University of Pennsylvania was the first American institution of higher education to offer a comprehensive curriculum in journalism, listing five courses in its 1893-94 catalog. Before the turn of the century, the University of Kansas, Denver University, Temple University, the University of Michigan, and the University of Nebraska had begun journalism instruction, in many instances as classes in English departments. By 1920, there were 131 colleges and universities teaching some journalism, and twenty-eight of these were giving professional courses.[13]

Still other developments indicated that journalism was becoming, in the words of E. L. Godkin, editor of the New York Evening Post, a "new and important calling."[14] In the 1870s and '80s, press clubs sprang up in New York, Minneapolis, St. Paul, Milwaukee, Boston, and San Francisco.[15] Professional journals appeared, the foremost being the Journalist, launched in 1884 and merged with Editor & Publisher in 1907.[16] Edwin L. Shuman's handbook for youths aspiring to newspaper careers, Steps into Journalism, was published in 1894, and a sequel, Practical Journalism, in 1903. Journalism, Shuman advised his readers, was a "profession requiring special training as imperatively as does that of medicine or the law."[17]

Despite acquiring some of the trappings of a profession, journalism alarmed the custodians of official culture. Newspapers were accused of everything from inciting crime and revolution to degrading the English language. A letter written to the Nation in 1903 charged that the popular press had contributed to the "prevailing spirit of lawlessness" in the country, "especially by sensationalism and by the reckless dissemination of false and pernicious ideas."[18] In 1909, the Century asserted, "The yellow journalist is becoming more audacious.... Where interviews cannot be had, they are sometimes obtained by extortion, under the threat of creating something seven times worse." And the magazine asked, "What is the use of pretending to a code of breeding and conduct, and of holding it up to one's children, if one admits into his home so insidious a foe as the yellow journal?"[19]

Such fulminations can be interpreted as further evidence of the newfound power of the press. To become the target of violent criticism, it was first necessary for journalists to achieve a degree of influence. Yet the attacks on their methods and mentality would eventually erode their self-image. Journalists would have their confidence in their work shaken. "Public acknowledgment of their prestige," Penn Kimball has pointed out, "is a sustaining element for those professions that have come to be 'recognized'."[20] Important segments of the public refused to acknowledge that there was anything prestigious about journalism. It was treated by the "better people" with bitter scorn. Behind the bravura of reporters who proclaimed themselves citizens of no mean state seethed self-doubt, self-doubt that would echo and reecho throughout the pages of newspaper fiction.

With the "new journalism" clamoring for attention and inciting moral controversy, public interest in the inner workings of the press was piqued. Shuman, in the Preface to his Practical Journalism, remarked, "There are few things concerning which the general public is more curious, and about which it knows less, than the inside of a metropolitan newspaper office."[21] It seems that like nature, authors of popular literature abhor a vacuum. Newspaper fiction arose partly in response to public curiosity about the big-city newspaperman who, supplied with a wad of copy paper, a stubby pencil, and a nose for news, had become by the 1890s an unmistakable figure on the American scene.

The potentially wide appeal of the genre was first demonstrated by Richard Harding Davis's "Gallegher, a Newspaper Story," the tale of a plucky copy boy who takes part in the capture of a notorious killer at a world-championship boxing match and then helps his Philadelphia paper scoop the competition with the news. Originally published in Scribner's Magazine in August 1890, "Gallegher" sold more than 50,000 copies when it appeared in book form, a not inconsiderable number for the time. Some later works of newspaper fiction also became best-sellers, Henry Sydnor Harrison's Queed in 1911 and both Katharine Brush's Young Man of Manhattan and Edna Ferber's Cimarron in 1930.

Whether best-selling or not, the fiction rarely rises above the puerile. Most of it has been forgotten because it is eminently forgettable. It wheezes and creaks with every shopworn device of sentimental literature. Courtship is idealized, and the last page of many novels features the chaste first kiss of the hero and heroine. There is an excess of plot as if to compensate for the lack of fully developed characters. The prose is sodden and gives off to the modern reader a mildewy smell.

Literary historian James D. Hart has noted that "the largest reading public of the years between the Spanish-American [War] and First World War insisted upon romance.... Confronted by a complex culture, depressed, confused, or yearning for a life happier than sober actuality, the people needed myths and symbols to endow them with strength and joy, and these they often found in the idyls of the printed page."[22] Changes in American society after World War I brought some changes in newspaper fiction, but not necessarily for the better. The most apparent was the open treatment of sex, encouraged by the popularization of Freudian psychology and the revolt of women against Victorian taboos. Male and female characters ceased to fumble, stammer, and blush in the presence of one another. Instead, they coupled like animals in heat or leeringly toyed with the possibility.

The prevailing cynicism of the Jazz Age filtered into newspaper fiction. A generation had, in F. Scott Fitzgerald's words, "grown up to find all Gods dead, all wars fought, all faiths in man shaken." Ben Hecht's Erik Dorn (1921) epitomized the new downbeat mood. "The rivers ... flow to the sea and life flows to death," Dorn declares with a sententiousness all too common among fictional journalists of the era. "And there is nothing else of consequence for intelligence to record."[23]

Of course, plenty of readers in the 1920s still exhibited a taste for chocolate-cream novels, and plenty of newspaper novels could still satisfy their craving. "Romance has always been an important element of America's popular literature," James D. Hart said, "for close adherence to fact or the exactitude of a reasoning mind set standards too demanding for a wide, democratic audience."[24] Awash in sentimentality when not dripping with cynicism, newspaper fiction routinely fails as art. The genre seems almost cursed. First-rate writers who tried their hands at it turned out second- and third-rate work.

Stephen Crane was hag-ridden by disease and debts when he wrote <u>Active Service</u>. Frank Norris had yet to embrace naturalism and was following in the romantic tradition of Robert Louis Stevenson and Rudyard Kipling when he wrote <u>Blix: A Love Idyll</u> (1899). Jack London had no excuse for "Amateur Night" (1903), whose title is an apt description of the quality of the story. It is an obvious piece of hack work. London knew that magazine editors would print practically anything with his name attached to it and ruthlessly traded on his reputation. He even evolved a philosophy of sorts to justify the prostitution of his talent. "If nothing goes with a name," he asked, "why strive?"[25]

Authors of far smaller ability than Crane, Norris, or London wrote most of the newspaper fiction published in the United States from 1890 to 1930. One might have expected them, nevertheless, to create a popular literature of some quality. The vast majority were journalists or former journalists, trained storytellers with inside knowledge of their subject. But the city rooms from which they graduated may have actually stultified their imaginations and warped their artistic judgment.

There is a legend that the city room is the place to begin if you want to learn to write. What Thomas Beer called the "romance of journalism as a school of letters" was well established by the 1890s.[26] It created a vortex that sucked into newspaper work such now-famous writers as Crane, Norris, Theodore Dreiser, and Ernest Hemingway. Their literary success, in turn, helped perpetuate the legend.

No other profession could match journalism for the variety and intensity of experience it offered aspiring authors in search of material. "The daily newspaper," reporter-turned-novelist David Graham Phillips said, "sustains the same relation to the young writer as the hospital to the medical student. It is the first great school of practical experience."[27] Examples abound of journalists who, having passed through the curriculum of the city room, graduated from journalism to literature. Among the first to do so was Richard Harding Davis. With the publication of "Gallegher" in 1890, the handsome, courtly Davis was dubbed the "American Kipling" and became the idol of newspapermen drudging on routine assignments and dreaming of better things.[28] John Dana, an executive on the <u>New York Sun</u>, said youths with literary ambitions

were eager to become reporters because Davis had begun
that way.[29]

Journalism and literature seemed to employ similar techniques and to have similar aims. "Writers of fiction are
spawned almost daily by the humbler press," H. W. Boynton
claimed in Atlantic Monthly in June 1904. "The journalistic
use of the word 'story' indicates the ease of a transition...."[30]
Thirty-six years later, Helen MacGill Hughes said, "Most reporters look upon themselves as novelists; they plan eternally
to write the great novel of the age."[31] Although the self-
image contained more than a trace of delusion, the comments
of one-time newspapermen continually propped it up. Maxwell
Anderson credited his reporting in San Francisco and New
York for his eventual success as a playwright. "I never completed a thing I wrote," he recalled, "until I learned to meet
the newspaper deadline."[32]

On the other hand, there were many who doubted the
value of journalistic experience in building a literary career.
"Such training," said Sinclair Lewis, who had worked briefly
for a paper in Cedar Rapids, Iowa, "is (always with exception) either useless or positively injurious." Lewis explained
that journalism teaches haste and fosters the habit of writing
under orders. Worse yet, it exposes one to "certain high-
lights of existence ... far less important to a genuinely creative writer than the steady, unmelodramatic daily life which
may be uninteresting as immediate news but which forms the
basis of all veritable poetry, fiction, or criticism."[33]

Journalist Richard Owen Boyer ridiculed the naiveté
of the cub reporter who thinks he will learn on a newspaper
how to write fiction. "The budding novelist," Boyer remarked in the American Mercury in January 1929, "finds out
that he cannot write, or if he can, that he won't, for newspaper men are primarily lazy and grow more lazy as the days
and years slip by."[34] The next month in the same magazine,
another journalist, Malvina Lindsay, warned that the "ambitious college graduate who enters a city room with a copy
of Proust under his arm soon discovers that legs are more
important in the newspaper business than any feeling for the
delicately turned phrase."[35]

Perhaps the strongest reservations about the usefulness
of journalistic training in achieving a literary career are found

in newspaper fiction. It is an ironic, but revealing, circum-
stance, since the fiction was written chiefly by men and
women who made the leap from journalism to literature.
"There are two kinds of newspapermen--" Chicago reporter
Ben Hecht observed in Erik Dorn, "those who try to write
poetry and those who try to drink themselves to death.
Fortunately for the world, only one of them succeeds."[36]
Katharine Brush, a former correspondent for the Boston
Traveler, displayed similar sarcasm in Young Man of Manhattan. The city room, she said, was "an excellent prep
school for writing; the trouble was you didn't graduate."[37]

Characters customarily distinguish between reporting
and writing. They disparage their journalism as "only a
trick," "scribble," "clever-silly" and "vaudeville."[38] Newspaper work causes them to squander their literary promise.
Condy Rivers, the protagonist of Frank Norris's Blix: A
Love Idyll, is cautioned by his girlfriend: "You've got it
in you ... to be a great story-teller.... But just so long
as you stay here [on a San Francisco daily], just so long
will you be a hack writer."[39]

Fictional reporters get conditioned to the peculiar
rhythms and requirements of journalism and flounder when
they attempt to write anything else. The heroine of Edna
Ferber's Dawn O'Hara (1911) complains:

> After working all day on a bulletin paper whose city
> editor is constantly shouting: "Boil it now, fellows!
> Keep it down! We're crowded!" it is too much of a
> wrench to find myself seated calmly before my own
> typewriter at night, privileged to write one hundred
> thousand words if I choose. I can't get over the
> habit of crowding the story all into the first para-
> graph. Whenever I flower into a descriptive passage
> I glance nervously over my shoulder, expecting to
> find Norberg stationed behind me, scissors and blue
> pencil in hand. Consequently, the book, thus far,
> sounds very much like a police reporter's story of a
> fire four minutes before the paper is due to go to
> press. [40]

It was more than journalism's quick, slick way of handling
material that could corrode creativity. The long, irregular
hours of newspaper work left little time or energy for serious

reading and writing. When Howard, the protagonist of
David Graham Phillips's The Great God Success (1901),
tries his hand at fiction, he finds that the "exactions of
newspaper life" have robbed him of strength for the effort.[41]

Equally crippling, their work set reporters oscillating
between the poles of cynicism and sentimentality. In their
restless search for the latest news, they became acquainted
with the night and deeds that required the cover of night.
"Doors opened at his knock," Stephen French Whitman said
of cub reporter Felix Piers in his 1910 novel, Predestined,
"and half-unwillingly, yet fascinated, he peered in at the
secret lives of strangers. He contemplated degradation; he
intruded on anguish; in awe he looked down at the mysteri-
ous masks of suicides and murdered men. He made the old
remark of all beginners in that business who are sensitive:
he had discovered the 'Human Comedy'--the comedy of human hearts, absurd, grotesque, repulsive, terrible."[42]
The young reporters went everywhere and witnessed everything, and soon they could believe in nothing and no one.

Their cynicism was a liability; it threatened to unfit
them for the "heart writing" cherished by newspapers.
This happens to Billy Woods, the protagonist of Jesse Lynch
Williams's "The Old Reporter" (1899), who "saw in a week
more bare reality, and more sorts of it, than most of you
run across in a year." Every passion and activity "had so
long ceased to mystify, charm, repell [sic] or awe him that
now he was forgetting how other people who had not lived
so fast were mystified, charmed, repelled, or awed." His
daily contact with tragedy, violence, and crime leads to a
"passive, premature mellowness" that cuts him off from the
human interest that is his stock in trade. "For Heaven's
sake," an editor tells him, "let up on those old worn-out
phrases. Get some new stencils."[43] Only sentimentality
could prevent journalists from disappearing under the weight
of their own cynicism. It was no accident that in the 1890s
there arose the stereotype of the "hard-drinking reporter who could talk with dry wit about the hundred and
one stiffs he had seen fished out of the river and shed
spontaneous tears over the urchin maimed by the passing
omnibus."[44]

Art, Flaubert said, "needs white, calm hands." Journalism molds life with nervous, ink-stained fingers into shrill

headlines and staccato stories. It may require either exceptional talent or exceptional luck to grow artistically amid the rush and strain of the city room. Lured into newspaper work by the hope that it will teach them to write, aspiring authors find themselves immured in a profession that prizes speed over deliberation, facileness over substance. Their imaginations, after chilling in the clichés of newswriting, may never completely thaw out.

As much as its themes, the shoddiness of most newspaper fiction points up the traumatic effects of journalistic experience on creative writers. The reporters-turned-novelists had passed through the news machine and been mangled. They followed artistic instincts that were wounded, futile, blind. The cheap finish and ready-made methods that characterized their journalism came to characterize their fiction as well.

That newspaper fiction is, on the whole, preposterously plotted and woodenly written should not automatically disqualify it from being studied.[45] Dorothy Burton Skaardal, a professor at the University of Oslo who uses American immigrant literature by Scandinavians as historical source material, suggested that "it is fairly easy for a person trained in literary criticism to separate out and discard those elements of fiction which are irrelevant to history.... What is of value to the historian in such works," she added, "is often present incidentally, even unconsciously: concrete detail, local color, attitudes revealed through authors' intrusive comments or slanted situations. Just who the hero is and who the villain can be significant, however wildly improbable the struggle between them."[46]

Newspaper fiction may seem a dubious place to explore journalism history, yet important clues to how journalists of the past felt about their work can be found there. Naturally, one cannot treat the fiction as if it were testimony given under oath. The novels and short stories deal in emotional, not literal, truth. But it is precisely this inner dimension that historians have had the greatest difficulty recapturing.

In the following pages, I trace the story patterns that run through forty years of newspaper fiction: the portrayal of journalism as either a school or a cemetery, the quest of the crusading journalist, and the idyll of country journalism.

Besides identifying the patterns, I try to place them within their historical contexts. Why, for example, did the journalist emerge as a crusader in newspaper fiction of the early 1900s? What was occurring in American society in general, and in journalism in particular, to generate the image? I also sketch, where possible, the journalistic backgrounds of the various authors. Many works of newspaper fiction are first novels, and, as is traditionally the case with such novels, they are heavily autobiographical.

I chose to concentrate on the period 1890-1930 in large part because technology and economics were transforming journalism from a craft into an industry throughout those years. Moreover, virtually every editorial device of the modern newspaper developed then, including the syndicated feature, comics, sports sections, Sunday supplements, and news photography. Journalism was gathering a mass audience, with the result that journalists inherited a wider and more controversial role in the life of the nation.

The 1890s represented a watershed not only in American journalism but also in American history. The decade saw the passing of the Old West, the shift of economic and political power from the countryside to the city, and the shattering impact of a torrent of immigration on traditional values and institutions. A series of violent strikes brought home to Americans the reality of class conflict, and the Spanish-American War awoke them to their responsibilities in world affairs. In the words of Henry Steele Commager, the nineties "fixed the pattern to which Americans of the next two generations were to conform, set the problems which they were required to solve."[47] The array of problems was bewildering. "My country in 1900," Henry Adams wrote, "is something totally different than my country in 1860.... Neither I, nor anyone else, understands it. The turning of a nebula into a star may somewhat resemble the change."[48]

A final reason for focusing on the period 1890-1930 is that after 1930, films began to supplant fiction as the leading popular art for portraying the press. There were several silent movies about journalism: Star Reporter (1921), Headlines (1925), and Freedom of the Press and Telling the World (both 1928). But, as Alex Barris observed in Stop the Presses!: The Newspaperman in American Films (1976),

"If there was ever any great (or even reasonably entertaining) silent newspaper movie it fails to come to mind." Sound provided the missing ingredient--dialogue--in 1929. "[A]lmost from the beginning of the talking area," Barris said, "the newspaperman has been a recognizable movie type, characterized by his wise-cracking, his insulting manner toward his bosses, and his breezy irreverence to editors, politicians, police, advertisers, publicity seekers, and female reporters."[49]

Clear parallels exist between newspaper fiction and newspaper films. The similarities can be explained by the fact that the films adopted unchanged the formulas that the fiction originated. Some movies were directly based on newspaper novels; Edna Ferber's Cimarron and Katharine Brush's Young Man of Manhattan were both made into films in 1930. Others were based on successful Broadway plays, such as Ben Hecht and Charles MacArthur's The Front Page and Louis Weitzenkorn's Five-Star Final. Because of the crossbreeding, the same stereotypes and story patterns appear in all the art forms. For example, the detective reporter is a stock character in fiction and on the stage and screen. Is it any wonder that one comes to side with the disgruntled cop in the film Deadline U.S.A. (1951) who asks, "When is the press going to grow up and stop playing detective?"

This study is organized thematically. Chapters II-IV are each devoted to a separate story pattern in newspaper fiction, which I have defined as any novel or short story with a journalist as the central character and journalism as at least a subplot. I examined seventy-eight of these works published in the United States from 1890 to 1930--and many more published later. I do not analyze them all individually; to have done so might have taxed the reader's patience beyond endurance. But all are there in the background shaping the discussion.

My concluding chapter investigates what newspaper fiction represented for its authors and readers and what it can represent for historians today. The relationship between art and life, Herbert J. Gans noted, "is very complex; sometimes one imitates another, but most often they travel along separate paths, with a variety of impacts on each other."[50] The public's fantasies and phobias about the press may have been played out in fiction. And real-life journalists may have patterned themselves to an extent on fictional models. With journalism schools and textbooks still scarce at the turn of the century, the young H. L. Mencken went to newspaper fiction for guidance once he had settled on a journalism career.[51] Uncounted others probably did the same. In the solitude of their secret hopes and fears, they may have clothed themselves in the fictional newspaperman's shiniest dreams and coffined themselves in his darkest nightmares.

## References

1. Quoted in Thomas Beer, Stephen Crane (New York: Knopf, 1923), p. 184.
2. George Santayana, "Justification of Art," Little Essays (New York: Scribner's, 1920), p. 112.
3. Frank Luther Mott, American Journalism, 3rd ed. (New York: Macmillan, 1962), p. 507.
4. Quoted in John Tebbel, The Life and Good Times of William Randolph Hearst (New York: Dutton, 1952), p. 79.
5. Quoted in Mott, American Journalism, p. 547.
6. Edward Alsworth Ross, "The Suppression of Important News," The Profession of Journalism, ed. by Willard Grosvenor Bleyer (Boston: Atlantic Monthly Press, 1918), p. 81.
7. Henry Steele Commager, The American Mind (New Haven: Yale University Press, 1950), p. 70.
8. Michael Schudson, Discovering the News (New York: Basic Books, 1978), p. 64.
9. Mott, American Journalism, p. 488.
10. Quoted in Allen Churchill, Park Row (New York: Rinehart, 1958), p. 224.
11. Julian Ralph, The Making of a Journalist (New York: Harper & Brothers, 1903), p. 27.
12. "Our Seventeenth 'Special,'" Journalist, Vol. 28, Dec. 15, 1900, p. 276.
13. Albert A. Sutton, Education for Journalism in the United States from Its Beginning to 1940 (Evanston, Ill.: Northwestern University Press, 1945), pp. 11, 17, 35.
14. Quoted in Schudson, Discovering the News, p. 70.
15. Ibid.
16. Mott, American Journalism, p. 490.
17. Edwin L. Shuman, Practical Journalism (New York: Appleton, 1903), p. 31.

18. "Newspaper Responsibility for Lawlessness," Nation, Aug. 20, 1903, p. 151.

19. "The Gentlemanly Reporter," Century, Nov. 1909, pp. 149-50.

20. Penn Kimball, "Journalism: Art, Craft or Profession?" in The Professions in America, ed. by Kenneth S. Lynn and the editors of Daedalus (Boston: Beacon Press, 1967), p. 243.

21. Shuman, Practical Journalism, p. vii.

22. James D. Hart, The Popular Book (Berkeley: University of California Press, 1963), p. 205.

23. Ben Hecht, Erik Dorn (New York: Putnam's, 1921; reprint ed., Chicago: University of Chicago Press, 1963), p. 344.

24. Hart, Popular Book, p. 205.

25. Andrew Sinclair, Jack: A Biography of Jack London (London: Weidenfeld & Nicolson, 1978), pp. 54-55, 77-78.

26. Beer, Stephen Crane, pp. 71-72.

27. Quoted in Larzer Ziff, The American 1890s (New York: Viking Press, 1968), p. 150.

28. Gerald Langford, The Richard Harding Davis Years: A Biography of a Mother and Son (New York: Holt, Rinehart & Winston, 1961), p. 114.

29. Fairfax Downey, Richard Harding Davis: His Day (New York: Scribner's, 1933), p. 79.

30. H. W. Boynton, "The Literary Aspects of Journalism," Atlantic Monthly, June 1904, p. 848.

31. Helen MacGill Hughes, News and the Human Interest Story (Chicago: University of Chicago Press; reprint ed., New Brunswick, N.J.: Transaction Books, 1981), p. 196.

32. Quoted in "Son Recalls Playwright Father," Grand Forks (N.D.) Herald, June 22, 1983, p. 1B.

33. Quoted in Silas Bent, Ballyhoo (New York: Boni & Liveright, 1927), pp. 112-13.

34. Richard Owen Boyer, "The Trade of the Journalist," American Mercury, Jan. 1929, p. 17.

35. Malvina Lindsay, "Jackdaw in Peacock's Feathers," American Mercury, Feb. 1929, p. 195.

36. Hecht, Erik Dorn, p. 20.

37. Katharine Brush, Young Man of Manhattan (New York: Farrar & Rinehart, 1930), p. 23.

38. David Graham Phillips, The Great God Success (New York: Grosset & Dunlap, 1901; reprint ed., Ridgewood,

N.J.: Gregg Press, 1967), p. 26; Olin L. Lyman, Micky (Boston: Richard G. Badger, 1905), p. 74; Floyd Dell, The Briary-Bush (New York: Knopf, 1921), pp. 168, 419.

39. Frank Norris, Blix: A Love Idyll, in A Novelist in the Making, ed. by James D. Hart (Cambridge: Belknap Press/Harvard University Press, 1970), pp. 208-9.

40. Edna Ferber, Dawn O'Hara (New York: Grosset & Dunlap, 1911), pp. 124-25.

41. Phillips, Great God Success, p. 32.

42. Stephen French Whitman, Predestined, with an afterword by Alden Whitman (New York: Scribner's, 1910; reprint ed., Carbondale: Southern Illinois University Press, 1974), pp. 56-57.

43. Jesse Lynch Williams, "The Old Reporter," The Stolen Story and Other Newspaper Stories (New York: Scribner's, 1899; reprint ed., Freeport, N.Y.: Books for Libraries Press, 1969), pp. 220-21, 248-49, 256-58.

44. Ziff, American 1890s, p. 153.

45. The little critical writing on newspaper fiction that exists is tendentious and superficial. I relied on none of it for my analysis, but I did find Thomas Elliott Berry's The Newspaper in the American Novel, 1900-1969 (Metuchen, N.J.: Scarecrow Press, 1970) useful for bibliographic purposes. The other works are:
Donna Born, "The Image of the Woman Journalist in American Popular Fiction, 1890 to the Present," paper presented to the Committee on the Status of Women of the Association for Education in Journalism, East Lansing, Mich., Aug. 1981;
Natalie F. Holtzman, "The Image of Women Journalists in the American Novel, 1898-1957," Matrix, Summer 1977, pp. 24-25, 31;
William McKeen, "Heroes and Villains: A Study of Journalists in American Novels Published between 1915 and 1975" (M.A. thesis, Indiana University, 1977).

46. Dorothy Burton Skaardal, "Immigrant Literature as Historical Source Material: Problems and Methods," paper presented to European Association for American Studies, Amsterdam, Netherlands, April 1980, p. 14.

47. Commager, American Mind, p. 53.

48. Quoted in Commager, American Mind, p. 134.

49. Alex Barris, Stop the Presses!: The Newspaperman in American Films (South Brunswick, N.J.: A. S. Barnes, 1976), p. 12.

50.   Herbert J. Gans, Popular Culture and High Culture (New York:   Basic Books, 1974), p. 14.
51.   H. L. Mencken, A Choice of Days, selected and with an introduction by Edward L. Galligan (New York: Vintage Books, 1981), p. 142.

Chapter II

## THE SCHOOL AND THE CEMETERY

This, then, had been his destiny from birth--
To desiccate life's pageant to a phrase--
Pity and terror, hunger, madness, mirth
Congealed in "Man Shoots Five in Murder Craze."
He'd written poems once.  He wrote no more.
His wits had chilled in stereotypes too long
To kindle now one glittering metaphor.
His pulse kept beat to headlines, not to song.
It was a sorry business, none knew better,
And there were moments when he was more than half
Persuaded to shrug loose the ultimate fetter ...
Save that he knew too well his epitaph,
And somehow could not stomach quite the crass
Brutality of "Scribe Ends Life With Gas."
                --Ted Olson

One occasionally encounters in newspaper fiction the notion
that the best reporters are born, not made.  Joseph A.
Altsheler, a former feature writer and editor on the New
York World, said in Gutherie of the Times (1904):  "There
are two kinds of correspondents; those who collect news
and those who absorb it.  Gutherie fell within the latter
class, which is by far the abler of the two, and know instinctively what things are worth."[1]

Most professional insiders, however, believed that a
nose for news is a hard-won acquisition rather than an
original trait of human nature.  "The only position that

occurs to me which a man in our Republic can successfully fill by the simple fact of birth," publisher Joseph Pulitzer wrote in 1904, "is that of an idiot."[2]  The conviction that special training is required for journalism is reflected in the titles that journalists gave their memoirs; for example, Julian Ralph's The Making of a Journalist (1903), Samuel Blythe's The Making of a Newspaper Man (1912), Will Irwin's The Making of a Reporter (1944), and Herbert L. Matthews' The Education of a Journalist (1956).

The chief plot of the newspaper fiction published from 1890 to 1930 dramatizes the belief that the cub reporter must be pushed, pounded, and pulled into shape.  It begins with a young, college-educated man entering journalism full of ideals and literary ambition and immediately suffering a series of humiliating setbacks.  His stories are either killed or cut beyond recognition.  He is snubbed by copy boys, abused by editors, and ignored by the rest of the staff. Then, just when he is about to be fired, he scores a sensational scoop and saves his job.  He has learned through bitter experience what makes a good story and a successful newspaperman.

After journalism has served him as a school, it may turn into a cemetery, to use David Graham Phillips's metaphor.  Newspaper work offers a smattering of all kinds of knowledge and can be used as a steppingstone to something else.  But the man who tries to make a career of it, who sticks to it, is doomed.  The protagonist listens to the cynical talk of veteran reporters and editors and sees the ruinous effects that long, irregular hours, low pay, and sordid prying into other people's affairs have had on them. Suddenly afraid for his future, he seeks to escape into a more rewarding and respectable line of work.

If he fails to get out, he ages prematurely.  His spirit slackens and sickens until he becomes a sad and frightening caricature of his younger self.  And when his usefulness is gone, he is tossed onto the scrap heap--a warning that the newspaper game may be too rough for those who try to play it.

Why journalism should be portrayed this pessimistically is a complex quesiton.  "No profession is so wept over," F. M. Colby said in the Bookman in 1902, adding that journalists themselves often shed the biggest tears.[3]  They are, by temperament and training, cavilers, constantly look-ing for things to criticize.  The story pattern embodies the revulsion of reporters-turned-novelists for the battering apprenticeship they were forced to endure in city rooms—and their criticism of the less talented men they left behind. "Journalism," observed Thomas Griffith, a former newspaper-man now with _Time_ magazine, "has always had a hard time of it among the literary, particularly among those who had to grub in it to enable them to write what they wanted to write, which society treated as a luxury when for them it was a necessity."[4]

Memoirs, handbooks, and trade magazines of the period referred to the lack of reward in journalism, but they did not dwell on it the way newspaper fiction does.  Still, the nonfiction provides clues to why the fiction denigrates news-paper work as a career.

Norman Hapgood, a reporter in Chicago, Milwaukee, and New York in the nineties before becoming editor of _Collier's_, said:  "In journalism men are likely to worsen as they grow older, and as they lose excitement.  There are not many pen-men who ... are most effective in old age."[5] Samuel Blythe noted that an "experienced doctor or an ex-perienced lawyer or an experienced banker gets better fees and is held in higher regard because of his experience" than an experienced newspaperman.  A reporter's greatest assets, Blythe lamented, "are youth and legs."[6]  The hope-lessness of the situation moved Charles Chapin, city editor of the _New York Evening World_, to remark of journalists, "The luckier ones die young."[7]

For the sensitive, the city room could be a torture chamber.  Edwin L. Shuman described the metropolitan news-paper office of the turn of the century as "neither a pure democracy nor a model republic, but an absolute despotism." Reporters lived in terror of "falling down" on an assignment and being summarily dismissed.  Rushing all over town after the latest news, then frantically churning out copy under deadline pressure, they soon burned out.  "Newspaper writ-ing," Shuman concluded, "in the essential qualifications required, is a learned profession; but in its exactions and its comparative insecurity it more nearly resembles a trade."[8]

Instead of admiring journalists for their hard work and dedication, publishers were contemptuous of them. James Gordon Bennett, Jr., owner of the New York Herald, never shook hands with an employee.[9] He used to boast, "I can hire all the brains I want for twenty-five dollars a week." Once, when Herald executives called a feature writer "indispensable," Bennett asked for a list of all the indispensable men on the staff. Then he fired them. "I will have no indispensable men in my employ," he explained to his secretary.[10]

Shortly after taking over the Herald from his father in 1868, Bennett devised a system of office spies. The tattletales were dubbed the White Mice because of their nibblings and squeakings. Joseph Pulitzer followed Bennett's example and established a similar network at the New York World.[11]

Frank A. Munsey promulgated oppressive office rules for the papers he published. The most infamous was the no-smoking rule at the Boston Journal, which Munsey bought in 1902. Finding clouds of tobacco smoke overhanging the city room and the back shop, the new owner declared: "I want notices put up, all around, 'No smoking.'... Do you know why I am stopping them from smoking? Whenever these men stop to puff a cigarette or light a pipe, they waste time. And God hates a waster." Munsey did not say whether God also hates fat men, but the cadaverous publisher clearly did, for he fired scores of them. In addition, he fired old men who showed their age and men who were untidy. One man even changed his name (Popp) because Munsey disliked the sound of it.[12]

Munsey owned a chain of grocery stores, and he brought the "grocery-chain theory" to journalism. "The same law of economics applies in the newspaper business that operates in all business today," he said. "Small units in any line are no longer competitive factors in industry, in transportation, in commerce, in merchandising and banking. Newspapers that disregard this economic law are inviting disaster...."[13] Munsey sold, bought, consolidated, and killed papers purely for profit. In doing so, he violated the romantic notion of reporters and editors that a newspaper was something "to be shaped into what they dreamed of by the care of their own hands, to be distinguished by their own taste and skill."[14] They feared and hated him for it.

Journalists were treated by publishers as hired men when they wanted to be treated as artists. The tension found its way into newspaper fiction and contributed to the portrayal of journalism as a cemetery. Another cause for the gloomy picture was the disdain of "respectable people" for yellow journals. "Everybody reads them," Whitelaw Reid told a lecture audience at Yale University in 1901, "and nearly everybody, among the more educated classes at least, abuses them."[15]

The eruption of yellow journalism was only one of many explosive changes that rocked the structure of American society in the eighties and nineties. Before 1880, the number of immigrants arriving in the United States reached 400,000 just once: in 1854. But in eight of the ten years after 1880, the total soared far above that figure.[16] The foreign-born crowded the cities, whose populations were further swelled by an exodus from the economically depressed Midwest. From 1890 to 1895, crop prices plunged, farm mortgages were foreclosed, and country banks shut their doors.

What are known as the Gay Nineties were not so very gay after all. The transition from the nineteenth to the twentieth century took place against a background of economic suffering and social unrest. In the spring of 1894, Coxey's army of unemployed marched on Washington. That summer, the Pullman strike in Chicago spread consternation and alarm. Its leader, Eugene Debs, was labeled an anarchist and imprisoned, and the federal government intervened with injunctions and troops.

If it was an especially bitter time for the poor, it was a time of almost unlimited opportunity for the moneyed. They learned from Darwin and Herbert Spencer that they were the fittest to survive, and they received assurance from Bishop Lawrence that "Godliness is in league with riches."[17] In 1895, the Supreme Court struck down the antitrust law and set the stage for the growth of monopolies, which gained control of natural resources, giant industries, and state legislatures through bribery and coercion.

The popular press both recorded and encouraged the metamorphosis of the United States from a nation of farms and small towns to one of factories and swarming cities. Yellow journalism was a product of, and participant in, the mechanization, urbanization, centralization, democratization, and vulgarization of culture. The cheap, mass-circulation dailies would have been unimaginable without factory girls and new immigrants to buy their sensational fare, or without such inventions as the telephone, typewriter, and Linotype to speed up production.

Yellow journals developed techniques peculiarly suited to the uncertain literacy of their audience and soon eclipsed the circulations of older, more staid papers. Joseph Pulitzer's New York World and William Randolph Hearst's New York Journal attracted laborers with crusades and sports pages, women with human-interest stories and advice columns, and immigrants with big pictures and one-syllable words. In playing up sex, crime, and violence, they built on precedents established by the penny press of the 1830s. The elder James Gordon Bennett launched the New York Herald as a one-cent daily in 1835 with the avowed purpose "not to instruct but to startle."[18]

Even so, yellow techniques were still novel enough in the mid-1880s to excite moral controversy. When the World ran a picture feature on the pretty girls of Brooklyn, reaction was swift and stinging. Angry Brooklynites threatened to horsewhip the scoundrels who had invaded their privacy, and Pulitzer's competitors took him to task for trampling on professional ethics. The Journalist editorialized, "It is just this sort of journalism that fosters [the idea] in the minds of the general public that a newspaperman has no conscience, and that when he enters the house it is a good time to lock up the spoons."[19]

Public officials resented the prying of the press no less than ordinary citizens did. The zeal of reporters in covering President Grover Cleveland's marriage and honeymoon in 1886 occasioned a national scandal. Cleveland flared out at "certain newspapers which violate every instinct of American manliness, and in ghoulish glee describe every sacred relation of private life."[20] Finley Peter Dunne, speaking through his fictional Irish barkeeper, Mr. Dooley, got it right: "They used to say a man's life was a closed book. So it is but it's an open newspaper."[21]

To the scared eyes of some, yellow journalists appeared to be children of the devil. E. L. Godkin, editor of the conservative <u>New York Evening Post</u>, condemned their work as "the nearest approach to Hell in any Christian state."[22] The Reverend Dr. W. H. P. Faunce, in a speech on the twenty-fifth anniversary of the New York Society for the Suppression of Vice in 1897, declared: "The press of this country to-day is engaged in a fearful struggle, one class against another. On one side stand the reputable papers which represent decency and truth, and on the other, is what calls itself the new journalism but which is in reality as old as sin itself."[23] The Newark public library and the Princeton Theological Seminary banned Pulitzer's and Hearst's papers, and leading men's clubs in New York stopped displaying them on tables.[24]

Such precautions proved futile in the end. The future drift of American journalism toward ever wider circulation through ever noisier appeals was already fixed. It might be, as Ambrose Bierce contended, that Hearst's sensational methods had "all the reality of masturbation."[25] But sensationalism met the needs and interests of the workers generated by industrial growth. Ill-educated, drudging in dull jobs, they were hungry for thrills. The tabloids that sprang into existence after World War I dragged the murky depths of the population for readers simply by updating, extending, and intensifying yellow techniques.

Yet those who were shocked and disgusted by sensationalism and the low-class audience it captured would get revenge. Yellow journals turned the custodians of official culture against the press as a whole, and the prejudice lingered a long time. As late as 1911, the <u>Outlook</u> was saying foreigners might be pardoned for thinking Americans "a race of moral degenerates." What else could they think, the magazine asked, when "sensational papers and many respectable journals as well devote more space to crime than to virtue and courage and honor, report at length the views of criminals and harlots, and invest lawbreakers with the interest and importance of great public figures"?[26] The "gutter journalism" of the tabloids set off a fresh round of attacks that lasted through the 1920s. In a typical diatribe, S. T. Moore branded the scandal sheets "an unholy blot on the fourth estate--they carry all the news that isn't fit to print."[27]

Under repeated barrages of criticism, reporters and

editors lost faith that journalism was a career worth pursuing. Theodore Dreiser came to feel while working for the
Chicago Globe and later for the St. Louis Globe-Democrat
that "the newspaper profession, the reporting end of it,
was the roughest, most degrading, most disheartening of
any.... Only the poor and outcasts seemed to stand in awe
of us, and not even those at times."[28] Nosey journalists
were viewed as perverts and parasites. The general lack
of respect gnawed at them. It induced insecurity about
their social status, and the insecurity is embodied--or, more
exactly, embalmed--in the portrayal of journalism as a cemetery.

Newspaper work might be arduous, unremunerative,
and disreputable, but college men, particularly the literary
sort, were drawn to it because it offered a chance to ac-
cumulate "experience." Richard Harding Davis said the cub
reporter "will find that he has crowded the experiences of
the lifetime of the ordinary young businessman, doctor, or
lawyer, or man about town, in three short years...."[29] The
city room was the greatest classroom in America. No other
occupation could approach journalism as a way to get to
know the world. Stanley Walker, city editor of the old
New York Herald Tribune, compared it to "some fabulous
university where the humanities are studied to the accompaniment of ribald laughter, the incessant splutter of an
orchestra of typewriters, the occasional clink of glasses,
and the gyrations of some of the strangest performers ever
set loose by a capricious and allegedly all-wise Creator."[30]

Fiction helped popularize the image of journalism as
a school. Ray Stannard Baker's short story "Pippins,"
published in the September 7, 1899, issue of Youth's Companion, is an early example. Baker graduated from Michigan Agricultural College (now Michigan State University)
and took additional courses at the University of Michigan,
including "Rapid Writing." Taught by English professor
Fred Newton Scott, it pioneered the study of journalism in
American colleges. In 1892, Baker, having decided on a
literary career, joined the reporting staff of the Chicago
Record. He had been there six years when he realized, as
he wrote his father in January 1898, that "newspaper work
would not do to grow old in...." Shortly after, he escaped
the rush and strain of daily journalism by accepting a job
with McClure's. His muckraking for the magazine in the

Progressive Era earned him the title "America's No. 1 Reporter."[31]

"Pippins" is what everyone in the city room of the Chicago Ledger calls James Northcote Lawrence, who is right out of college and "beaming with confidence in himself." But the cub soon has his confidence rattled. Writing up a fire one night, Pippins is "keenly conscious of his college Latin and French" and sprinkles "a metaphor here and a simile there, to make the story sparkle...." The next morning, he is surprised not to see his effort on the front page—or on the second or third. He finds it buried in the back of the paper, his literary flourishes "remorselessly cut out."[32]

Before he can succeed in newspaper work, Pippins must have the "college" knocked out of him. He must shed his educated—that is, false and effeminate—ideas. Only then will he be ready to prove that he has the makings of a journalist.

His big break comes one blustery December night when he is sent to discover why the men at a waterworks intake crib on Lake Michigan have run up a distress flag. Under trying conditions, he gathers the facts, and after the tugboat captain who took him to the island refuses to leave because of ice on the lake, he sets out for shore on foot. He crashes through the ice, but "spurred by the thought of a beat," saves himself from drowning.[33]

Although soaked and shivering, Pippins hurries straight to the office to write his account. He forgets in his excitement "all his Latin and French" and tells "the story as it happened in crisp, short sentences." He scoops even "the great Keenan" of the rival Times, "who had been through half a dozen Indian wars and had brought back a long jagged scar on one cheek as a souvenir of one of them." The Ledger's city editor says simply, "You'll do, Pippins." Journalism being an unpretentious, common-sense business, this bald remark is "the greatest praise that ever comes to a newspaper man."[34]

In "Pippins," as in most newspaper fiction, a college degree is worse than useless; it is an actual hindrance to the young reporter. Baker's story reflects a longstanding belief in the superiority of practical experience to formal education. Frederic Hudson, editor of the New York Herald, voiced the prevailing view when he said in 1875: "The only place where one can learn to be a journalist is in a great newspaper office.... College training is good in its way, but something more is needed for journalism."[35] Many of the successful editors of the era had begun as printer's devils or copy boys and worked their way up. They saw little reason to doubt the soundness of their training in the "school of hard knocks."

On the surface, paradoxically, newspaper fiction seems to repudiate the traditional prejudice against book learning. By regularly portraying old newspapermen as cynics, rummies, and hacks, it creates the impression that the influx of college graduates into city rooms in the 1890s was ushering in a golden age of journalism. Richard Harding Davis claimed in "The Reporter Who Made Himself King" (1891) that it was a disadvantage to start out as a copy boy who, in Horace Greeley's phrase, "slept on newspapers and ate ink"[36]:

> Now, you cannot pay a good reporter for what he does, because he does not work for pay. He works for his paper. He gives his time, his health, his brains, and his sleeping hours, and his eating hours, and sometimes his life, to get the news for it. He thinks the sun rises only that men may have light by which to read it. But if he has been in a newspaper office from his youth up, he finds out before he becomes a reporter that this is not so, and loses his real value. He should come right out of the University where he has been doing "campus notes" for his college weekly, and be pitchforked out into city work without knowing whether the Battery is at Harlem or Hunter's Point, and with the idea that he is a Moulder of Public Opinion and that the Power of the Press is greater than the Power of Money, and that the few lines he writes are of more value in the Editor's eyes than is the column of advertising on the last page, which they are not.[37]

Cubs instinctively shrink from newspaper veterans as from death's-heads. The protagonist of Wayland Wells Williams's Goshen Street (1920) was

repelled by their unattractive appearance, their
heavy badinage, their noisy excursions to the bar;
he noticed two or three of them were gray-haired
men of fifty and became afraid. What if _he_ should
degenerate into that distressing product, the elderly
reporter, being sent out on less and less important
stories, trying to belie his failure by boasting of
past triumphs?[38]

But such fear and disgust tend to be tempered by the dy-
namics of the plot. It develops that the secrets to success
in newspaper work are stored in the whisky-addled brains
of the old-timers. "When you are done with me," declares
one who has taken the young hero of Edward Hungerford's
The Copy Shop (1925) under his wing, "you can forget all
that journalism stuff they tried to teach you in that fresh-
water college of yours. I am going to show you the real
thing."[39]

Linton, the protagonist of Jesse Lynch Williams's
"The New Reporter" (1899), cannot adjust to the sordid-
ness of the "real thing" without an inner struggle. Williams
was a product of Princeton and the New York Sun. At the
turn of the century, the Sun was known as "the newspaperman's newspaper," where stylish writing was recognized and
encouraged. A former star reporter on the paper, Will Irwin, said, "it was no accident that the Sun, both morning
and evening, was in that period the most prolific feeder of
American literature."[40] Besides Williams, authors of newspaper fiction who worked for it included Richard Harding
Davis, David Graham Phillips, Samuel Hopkins Adams, Irvin
S. Cobb, and Stephen French Whitman.

Like Pippins, Linton thinks his college background
will enable him to master journalism with relative ease. He
is chagrined to discover that "Not even William Shakespeare
would know what to get or how to put it without some training at reporting." The bumbling cub is "bossed around and
jumped upon and made to feel very small and stupid and in
the way." He tolerates the abuse because newspaper work
acquaints him with humanity as no other course of instruction
can. At school, he read "theories of man as a unit," but
now he encounters "men as warm human beings, with their
passions and pursuits, their motives and their way of looking
at things."[41]

Exciting and interesting as Linton's job is, he is disturbed by certain demands it makes on him. He finds it "sort of hard on one's self-respect," for example, to ask a red-eyed widow if it is true her husband was a drunk. Until he loses his fastidiousness about "talking to people about things they did not want to talk about," he is a failure as a reporter. He finally argues himself into believing that "news was a commodity and that there was just as much dignity in the getting, handling, selling of it as of woolens or professional opinion or any other article of merchandise." After overcoming the twin handicaps of higher education and middle-class morality, he is given his own writing table, "with as many cockroaches in the drawers as any of the tables...."[42] Williams agreed with Baker that college training could hold back a cub, but at least he had the good grace to be somewhat ironic about it.

Theodore Dreiser, in his collection Free and Other Stories (1918), depicted the dilemma of a college-educated reporter who refused to shed his college ways. Dreiser had a lot of naive ideas about journalism before he entered the field. "Because newspapers were always dealing with signs and wonders, great functions, great commercial schemes, great tragedies and pleasures," he recalled, "I began to conceive of them as wonderlands in which all concerned were prosperous and happy. I painted reporters and newspaper men generally as receiving fabulous salaries, being sent out on the most urgent and interesting missions. I think I confused ... reporters with ambassadors and prominent men generally."[43]

In 1892, Dreiser was hired by the Chicago Globe. Five months later, already a star reporter, he joined the St. Louis Globe-Democrat. His false romanticism had given place to cynical knowledge. "[T]he daily routine of my work," he explained, "seemed to provide ample proof that life was grim and sad. Regularly it would be a murder, a suicide, a failure, a defalcation which I would be assigned to 'cover,' and this would be contrasted on the same day, say, with an important wedding, a business or political banquet, a ball or club entertainment of some kind, which would provide just the necessary contrast to prove that life was haphazard and cruel; to some lavish, to others not so."[44] There is significance in the fact that the pioneer realists of American literature--Dreiser, Stephen Crane, Frank Norris,

and David Graham Phillips—all passed through journalism.
As young reporters, they got an unforgettable close-up
view of the new America: the sweatshops and grimy factories, the hordes of immigrants, the big-city slums and
strikes, and the wealth and poverty side by side.

Dreiser's "A Story of Stories," while written in a humorous mock-heroic style, is vicious in its implications. It
focuses on the rivalry between "Red" Collins, a "slithery,
self-confident" police reporter with a taste for loud clothes
and a distaste for would-be writers, and Augustus Binns,
"rather graceful as college men go, literary of course, highly ambitious, with gold eye-glasses, a wrist watch, a
cane...." The shrewd, ruthless Collins scoops the educated, effete Binns, who can only wonder: "Am I really
the lesser and this scum the great? Do writers 'grow on
trees'?"[45] College training and artistic temperament are
shown to be inadequate when pitted in the newspaper arena
against experience and animal cunning. Too much education
leaves the reporter out of touch with the real world. In
such an eminently practical field as journalism, the lower
your intellect and aspirations, the better.

And yet "Nigger Jeff," another story in the collection,
suggests that journalism can be an excellent prep school for
writing, if the student is willing to learn. Reporter Elmer
Davis is a "vain and rather self-sufficient youth who is in-
clined to be of that turn of mind which sees in life only a
fixed and ordered process of rewards and punishments."[46]
Davis receives an out-of-town assignment that puts his as-
sumptions to the test. He is sent to cover the lynching of
a black man accused of raping the nineteen-year-old daughter of a rich white farmer.

The nearer he gets to the site of the trouble, the
ironically named village of Pleasant Valley, the more agitated
Davis becomes. "In his fixed code of rewards and punishments he had no particular place for lynchings.... It was
too horrible a kind of reward or punishment." But once he
arrives, he manages to suppress his misgivings, and when
the lynch mob drags the black man from the sheriff's house,
he is "eager to observe every detail of the procedure." He
carefully notes the "color values" of the shocking scene:
"the red, smoky heads of torches, the disheveled appearance
of the men, the scuffling and pulling."[47]

Later, Davis visits the dead man's shack. While sur-
veying the corpse, whose bier is an ironing board, he is
startled by a "half sigh, half groan." He notices for the
first time an old woman weeping in a dark corner. "Before
such grief his intrusion seemed cold and unwarranted."[48]
He withdraws, tears burning his eyes.

Gradually, he regains his composure and, "with the
cruel instinct of the budding artist," begins to "meditate
on the character of the story he would make.... The knowledge now that it was not always exact justice that was meted
out to all and that it was not so much the business of the
writer to indict as to interpret was borne in on him." Already sifting and connecting the kaleidoscopic images of the
night, Davis exclaims, "I'll get it all in."[49]

Helen MacGill Hughes said in News and the Human Interest Story that journalism develops in the reporter an
"aloofness from personal passion that, in one direction,
marks the case-hardened cynic, and, in the other, the
philosopher and artist."[50] Davis realizes he must control
his feelings so he can concentrate on observing and de-
scribing. He is shaken by what he sees, but as a hired
spectator, he cannot follow his natural impulse to act in an
emergency. Journalism trains him to distance himself from
raw experience and distill it with clinical detachment into
the stuff of art.

So far, I have dealt only with short stories that portray journalism as a school. There were also several novel-
length treatments of the theme. The most popular--and,
of course, worst written--was Queed by former Richmond,
Virginia, newspaperman Henry Sydnor Harrison. Published
on May 6, 1911, this incredible tale of a homely, arrogant
young intellectual who is transformed by love into the handsome, successful editor of a Southern daily caught the public fancy. Readers in need of a sugar fix bought 400,000
copies, enough to make Harrison's first novel the number
four best-seller of the year.[51]

A more distinguished first novel, Meyer Levin's Reporter, met a less distinguished fate. Not long after it appeared in 1929, its publisher suppressed it because a news-
paperwoman who thought it maligned her threatened to
sue.[52] That was unfortunate, for the book was written in

a bold, inventive style, a volatile mixture of journalese and
Joycean stream of consciousness.

The feverish, fragmented prose is meant to convey
the breakneck pace of Chicago journalism, in which Levin
had worked on and off for five years. In the following
passage, the protagonist, a college-trained cub, is trying
to get information about the girlfriend of murdered policeman
Walter Ryan:

> Luck. They know. Girl's name Bella Morris
> lives at--
> Phone in girl's name, address. Where the hell's
> a car line now. Where the hell can you get a cab
> in this tail's end; he gets a car and flops off into
> a cab. Girl's home. Picture? Picture? Her thin-
> eyed father is quiet in the kitchen. Yes, he sober-
> ly says, she's heard about the shooting and she's
> gone to the hospital now. Yes, they were to have
> been married.
> Please, please. Picture of hero's grieving
> sweetheart. No picture.
> Off quick to Ryan's house....[53]

To illustrate the bizarre antics and crude appeals that
tabloids of the twenties used to boost circulation, Levin reproduced scareheads at the top of each page: "AUTOS KILL
SEVEN IN DAY," "WOULD HAVE SELF SHOT TO MARS,"
"RIPPER ATTACKS GIRL." For the same reason, he also
scattered "hot" stories in long, narrow newspaper columns
throughout the narrative. Some of the stylistic fireworks
fizzle and pop rather than whiz and bang, but the overall
effect is spectacular. The wild, irresponsible world of sensational journalism is noisily lit up.

Levin's protagonist is called simply "the reporter,"
and he is the stereotypical cub of fiction. He is Ray Stannard Baker's Pippins and Jesse Lynch Williams's Linton re-
incarnated. His anxieties and ambitions are theirs carried
forward into the Jazz Age.

Journalism offers him a more valuable education than
the one he received at college. The lessons can be stomach-
churning, as when he watches an autopsy on a bullet-
riddled gangster. But they always demand his full attention

--and usually repay it. Sent on a story, he must keep his senses on "red alert" so as not to miss any important details. "He notices, notices everything."[54]

The reporter has moments of rebellion against the crassness of journalism: "Out, out, seek air, seek change! He was certainly weary of this tawdry newspaper game. No chance of artistic expression."[55] Although he daydreams of becoming a painter, a movie star, a novelist, that is as close as he ever comes to quitting. At the end, he is still the quintessential cub, chasing the latest sensation, racing the next deadline--and wondering why.

Other protagonists do flee the daily grind. They get an education and get out. If they stay on newspapers, they are doomed. Time and the current of news running through them burn out their interest in what they see and tell. "Journalism is not a career," a disillusioned reporter asserts in David Graham Phillips's The Great God Success. "It is either a school or a cemetery. A man may use it as a stepping-stone to something else. But if he sticks to it, he finds himself an old man, dead and done for to all intents and purposes before he's buried."[56]

The price of an education comes high. In "The Reporter Who Made Himself King," Richard Harding Davis wrote that the cub discovers after three years--"it is sometimes longer, sometimes not so long"--that "he has given his nerves and his youth and his enthusiasm in exchange for a general fund of miscellaneous knowledge...."[57] Linton is the exception that proves the rule; despite working at all hours, in all kinds of weather, and seeing all sorts of things, his health holds up. As Williams explained, "On The Day they used to reckon on cubs breaking down at some stage of the first year or so; then, if they don't die, they are supposed to have their second wind after that, and to keep in fairly good health if they leave whisky alone."[58]

Old reporters traditionally lift a warning hand to those entering journalism. "There's no future for a man in the newspaper business," one cautions in Ben Ames Williams's Splendor (1927). "Nothing but a lot of work and a sanitarium when your nerves play out. Late hours, long hours, dull scratching at things."[59] Another tells the hero of Malcolm H. Ross's Penny Dreadful (1929): "Leave the game

before you are forced out of it."[60]   Not all need to be told.
A number recognize in the beaten look and cynical talk of
veteran newspapermen damning evidence that journalism de-
vours its young.   "I don't want to burn out in this business," says the protagonist of Gene Fowler's Trumpet in the
Dust (1930).   "They use you until you are all consumed and
then toss you aside like a handful of wet ashes."[61]

Thus, newspapers lose their slaves.   Most go into lit-
erature.   Condy Rivers in Frank Norris's Blix:   A Love
Idyll (1899), Joe Blake in George Cary Eggleston's Blind
Alleys (1906), and Toby McLean in Katharine Brush's
Young Man of Manhattan (1930) are examples.   Some, such
as John Harkless in Booth Tarkington's The Gentleman from
Indiana (1899), Billy Gutherie in Joseph A. Altsheler's
Gutherie of the Times (1904), and Jeremy Robson in Samuel
Hopkins Adams's Common Cause (1919) go into politics.
And a few--Lawrence Ashmore in Charles Agnew McLean's
The Mainspring (1912) is one--go into business.   But which-
ever path they take, they flee down it just as fast as they
can.

The killing effects of journalism, and the struggle to
escape them, are depicted in Edna Ferber's first novel,
Dawn O'Hara.   Dawn is that rare specimen in newspaper
fiction:   the female protagonist.   The vast majority of central characters are men because the newspaper was, as Edwin L. Shuman put it, "distinctively a masculine institution
offering women ... the frills and fringes of journalistic
work."   It was felt that "a girl can not live in the free-
and-easy atmosphere of the local room or do the work required of a reporter without undergoing a decline in the
innate qualities of womanliness and suffering in health."
At the turn of the century, Edward M. Bok of the Ladies
Home Journal asked fifty male editors and fifty newspaper-
women whether they would want a daughter of theirs to enter journalism.   The responses to the survey are revealing.
Forty-two women answered--three yes and thirty-nine no.
Thirty men answered--all no.[62]

Both male and female reporters in fiction are likely
to grow disenchanted, but since women were considered
frailer and more emotional, their disenchantment is magnified
and speeded up.   A sob sister in Brander Matthews's "An
Interview with Miss Marlenspuyk" (1895) decides to quit her

job after a single conversation with an old maid who says she would sooner survive on "cold water and a dry crust" than earn her living as a yellow journalist.[63]  In Elizabeth G. Jordan's "Miss Van Dyke's Best Story" (1898), a reporter finds her forays into sensational journalism have soiled her reputation among the men on the staff.  They begin treating her as "one of themselves, with a good-natured camaraderie...."[64]  Instead of being pleased at the equal treatment, she is alarmed and offended to be no longer placed on a pedestal and leaves the paper to get married.

Dawn O'Hara portrays journalism with a curious combination of fondness and fear.  Ferber, who worked for the Appleton (Wis.) Crescent and the Milwaukee Journal, did not like the novel when she completed it so she threw it away.  Her mother rescued the manuscript and sent it to a publisher, and it appeared in 1911.[65]

The book opens with Dawn, a reporter on a New York daily, hospitalized for nervous exhaustion.  Her husband, also a reporter, is in even worse shape.  He had been the most brilliant writer on the paper--and the most dissolute. When his benders became too frequent, he was replaced by a man less brilliant but more dependable.  His firing pushed him over the edge into madness, and he has been confined in an asylum for years.

Like an addiction to heroin, journalism is a hard-to-break habit with catastrophic consequences.  While recuperating at her married sister's home in northern Michigan, Dawn indicates that she plans to return to newspaper work once she is well.  She sounds almost helpless to resist the urge to plunge back into the pandemonium of the city room:

> After you have been a newspaper writer for seven years--and loved it--you will be a newspaper writer, at heart and by instinct at least, until you die. There's no getting away from it.  It's in the blood. Newspaper men have been known to inherit fortunes, to enter politics, to write books and become famous, to degenerate into press agents and become infamous, to blossom into personages, to sink into nonentities, but their news-nose remained a part of them, the inky, smoky, stuffy smell of a newspaper was ever sweet in their nostrils.[66]

The allure of journalism is that it offers experience in a hurry. "I have come to the conclusion," Dawn says, "that one year of newspapering counts for two years of ordinary existence, and that while I'm twenty-eight in the family Bible I'm fully forty inside." With wider experience than the average woman, she is "spoiled for sewing bees and church sociables and afternoon teas."[67]

Yet Dawn senses that the excitement of reporting is largely an illusion. The atmosphere of rush and strain obscures how hollow the rewards of newspaper work really are. "We contrive and scheme and run about all day getting a story," she observes. "And then we write it at fever heat, searching our souls for words that are clean-cut and virile. And then we turn it in, and what is it? What have we to show for our day's work? An ephemeral thing, lacking the first breath of life; a thing that is dead before it is born."[68]

Deep as her doubts about journalism are, Dawn takes a job on the Milwaukee Post when she recovers from her breakdown. Her husband, released from the asylum, follows her there. His threatening behavior toward her shows he is still unbalanced. According to the laws of popular fiction, he must be punished for his brutality and madness, and he dies in a car crash. Dawn is free, finally, to marry her doctor. Perhaps she would have slipped from newspaper bondage anyway. She has had a novel accepted for publication and is ready to graduate to literature. It was a measure of Ferber's own anxiety about escaping the city room that she provided Dawn with a couple of clearly marked exits.

Not everyone gets out alive. The city room is a cemetery for some. They die, either literally or figuratively, as a result of the wounds inflicted by daily journalism. Billy Woods, the protagonist of Jesse Lynch Williams's "The Old Reporter" (1899), is pulverized in the "great, all-devouring machine that turns out the stuff called news." Friends on the New York Day, foreseeing what will happen, urge him to write books or work for a magazine or go into politics. But he ignores their advice. "It's the only way to live," he says of reporting. "I expect to die out on a story." And emotionally, he does. He sees so much that his personal zest in seeing things wears out. His copy becomes stale. He tries to pour sparkle and human interest

back into it by means of a few drinks snatched between assignments. Before long, he is an alcoholic, unable to hold
a steady job. He ends as one of the "ghosts of Printing
House Square," living on memories and the money he can
cadge from former colleagues.[69]

Stephen French Whitman's naturalistic novel Predestined vividly unfolds the chief story pattern of newspaper
fiction from school to cemetery. The crucial phase of
America's first full-scale literary war was waged in the
1890s. On one side were the realists; on the other, the
romanticists. Battle was joined over the question of whether
literature should portray shameful and ugly facts or, for
the sake of decency, varnish, veil, and perfume them. It
was an era of startling disparities, of vast fortunes piled
up by robber barons amid unemployment, pauperism, and
starvation. Writers were choosing, in effect, between social realism and social romanticism, between political reform
and the political status quo. With Hamlin Garland, Stephen
Crane, Frank Norris, and Theodore Dreiser forming the
shock troops, realism won a place in American letters by
the close of the nineteenth century, though sharp skirmishes
continued to be fought.[70]

Predestined is a link in the development of American
realistic fiction from Norris, Dreiser, and the rest of their
depressing band to Sinclair Lewis, F. Scott Fitzgerald, and
Ernest Hemingway. Whitman, who had been a reporter on
the New York Evening Sun for four years, published the
book about a month after his thirtieth birthday. In time,
it gathered a cult following. Fairfax Downey quoted admir-
ingly from it in his 1933 biography of Richard Harding
Davis. More impressively, Fitzgerald proposed in a letter
to Charles Scribner in 1922 that his publishing house bring
out a Scribner library and that it include Whitman's first
novel.

"Take for instance Predestined and The House of
Mirth," Fitzgerald wrote. "I do not know, but I imagine
these books are kept upstairs in most bookstores, and only
obtained when someone is told of the work of Edith Wharton
and Stephen French Whitman. They are almost as forgotten
as the books of Frank Norris and Stephen Crane were five
years ago, before Boni's library began its career." Of the
eighteen books he recommended for a Scribner library,

Fitzgerald ranked <u>Predestined</u> second, after <u>The House of Mirth</u> or <u>Ethan Frome</u>. He ranked his own <u>This Side of Paradise</u> third.[71]

Whitman's protagonist, Felix Piers, starts out as a young man of literary promise and social position and decays into a derelict who kills himself. Felix comes to ruin through the complex interplay of hereditary and environmental forces. He is the victim of a volatile temperament, unfortunate love affairs, and the poisonous atmosphere of big-city newspapers.

After graduating from college, Felix becomes enflamed with literary ambition. An established novelist advises him that journalism provides ideal training for literature. Felix applies for a reporting job on the <u>New York Evening Sphere</u>. "I'm doing it because I want to learn to write good English," he tells the editor, who hires him at $15 a week.[72]

As a member of the "fraternity of young men who hurry forth throughout the city at the first hint of unusual happenings," Felix gets an education. He learns about the human comedy: "absurd, grotesque, repulsive, terrible."[73] The awful knowledge burns out his enthusiasm, and he pines for his apprenticeship in the shabby newspaper office to end.

Meanwhile, his private life is crumbling. His engagement to the daughter of an old, wealthy New York family breaks up after he has an affair with his best friend's wife. He drinks, resolves to stop, and fails to keep his resolutions.

His troubles outside work only increase his loathing for work. "Climbing the spiral staircase, emerging into the office of <u>The Evening Sphere</u>, to be enveloped invariably by the same pandemonium, he felt as if he were slipping into one of those confused dreams full of interminable, distasteful labors." Finally, on the strength of a few published short stories, he quits. He is too occupied with visions of literary success to "think of writing murder stories" for a newspaper anymore.[74]

Success never materializes. He has another self-destructive romance. On the rebound from it, he marries an emotionally unstable woman. His drinking accelerates.

Penniless, he pawns his jewelry, borrows money from friends with no hope of repaying it, and then returns in humiliation to the Sphere.

Where Felix once considered himself above newspaper work, he now is barely able to perform it. He views assignments that take him out of the office as opportunities to "snatch some highballs." The editor no longer trusts him with sensitive stories that could involve the paper in libel suits. He is shifted to the copy desk, "journalism's Boot Hill."[75]

Worse is still to come. When the Sphere's owner orders economies, Felix is fired. His wife dies, and though their marriage was miserable, he is devastated. He drifts onto the staff of the Torch, a yellow journal whose cynical sensationalism--"accuracy was a negligible quality; mendacity which produced a thrill was an accomplishment"--parallels his own spiritual squalor.[76] He is fired without warning from the Torch, too.

Desperate for money, he turns to writing scenarios for silent movies. "He dismissed from his mind his last aspirations toward subtlety, poetry, and technical excellence in exposition; he invited, instead, those motives of inordinate heroism, villainy, and self-sacrifice ... so satisfactory to the leaders of dull lives, who ... glimpse in the feverish atmosphere of protagonists exquisitely valiant and magnanimous, something of their own secret longings."[77] Predestined offers no idealized hero or happy ending to touch up unpleasant reality. Its protagonist, dragged down by drunkenness and despair, commits suicide with an overdose of sleeping powders.

Whitman's portrayal of journalism as a cemetery was far from unique. Many a city room in fiction contains walking corpses, and many a cub reporter gags on the smell of death and decay. But most cubs get out, through one authorial contrivance or another, before they are fatally contaminated. Whitman leaves Felix to rot and records his decomposition in all its horror. Predestined bravely pointed toward the more truthful treatment of material that would mark American literature following World War I.

The 1920s, which brought speakeasies, collegiate

whoopee, big-time sports, and movie-star worship, have
been dubbed the Age of Wonderful Nonsense. Released
from the sacrifice and strain of war, Americans sought entertainment and escape. Their headlong pursuit of thrills
partly concealed their disillusionment with the social order
of the day. Below the surface, a fateful change was taking
place, the result of the war, Prohibition, the automobile,
the assembly line, the agitation of women for the vote and
careers, the new and disturbing findings of science, and
the revolt of youth against Victorian taboos. The majority
of Americans, Frederick Lewis Allen said, "felt a queer dis-
appointment after the war, they felt life was not giving them
all they hoped it would, they knew that some of the values
which once meant much to them were melting away...."[78]

Millions of people were moving toward the bon vivant's
idea of proper morality: "A single standard, and that a
low one."[79] Freudian psychology, as popularized by magazines and newspapers, taught that it was unhealthy to deny
sexual drives. Supposedly nice girls wore lipstick and
rouge, smoked cigarettes, and drank cocktails. The liber-
ated moral code of the younger generation filtered into literature. Authors approached sex with an openness that
was revolutionary. In the newspaper fiction of the decade,
protagonists were as randy as their forerunners were re-
pressed.[80] "When strongly sexed men fought against desire, it made them sick, melancholy, fanatical," Gene Fowler
wrote in Trumpet in the Dust to justify his hero's dalli-
ances.[81]

Fictional newspapermen were still tormented, only they
were not tormented by sexual frustration. Their anxiety
reflected that of America, vaguely yearning for something
more. It also reflected the vicious attacks on journalism
provoked by the circus antics of tabloids.

Joseph Medill Patterson's New York Illustrated Daily
News, the first tabloid in the United States, appeared on
the morning of June 26, 1919, two days before the signing
of the Treaty of Versailles. Its heavy use of photographs,
its bold treatment of sensational subjects, and its lotteries,
giveaways, and other promotional gimmicks found a waiting
audience. By 1924, the Daily News (Illustrated had been
dropped from its name) had a circulation of 750,000, the
largest in the nation, and the figure reached 1.32 million
by 1929.[82]

The success of the Daily News inspired dozens of
imitators. Tabloids spread over the country, answering
the same need for excitement and distraction as marathon
dancing, flagpole sitting, and other phenomena of the twenties. "Ours is a restless populace," Silas Bent noted in
1927, "handcuffed to a mechanical monotony and ever atiptoe
for another thrill. In a channel swimmer, a bathing beauty,
a tennis player, a pugilist, a motion picture star, it may
find vicarious escape from the commonplace of machinery;
and the newspaper undertakes profitably to provide the
escape."[83]

Despite--or, perhaps, because of--its popularity,
tabloid journalism was attacked by the custodians of official
culture. The charges hurled at it were reminiscent of those
hurled at yellow journalism in the 1880s and 1890s. Abel
Kandel complained in the Forum that the tabloid "reduced
the highest ideals of a newspaper to the process of fasten-
ing a camera lens to every boudoir keyhole."[84] But vul-
garity was by no means its exclusive property. The entire
press had been, in Bent's words, "tarred with the stick of
the tabloid, tarred with its pictures, its headlines, its sensationalism, its rowdyism, its meddlesomeness."[85] Fiction
had always darkly mirrored the doubtful status of journalists in American society, and the darkness grew as all of
journalism suffered a loss of prestige in the furor over the
tabloids.

Ben Hecht's first novel, Erik Dorn (1921), is typical
of the gloomy newspaper fiction that came out of the Jazz
Age: Floyd Dell's Moon-Calf (1920) and The Briary-Bush
(1921), Heywood Broun's The Boy Grew Older (1922), Harvey Fergusson's Capitol Hill (1923), Grove Wilson's Man of
Strife (1925), and Malcolm H. Ross's Penny Dreadful (1929).
Hecht was only sixteen when he broke into big-city reporting in 1910. He and the other "kid reporters" on the
Chicago Journal carried their responsibilities lightly. They
considered journalism "some sort of game like stoop-tag."[86]

After four years, Hecht switched to the Chicago Daily
News. Harry Hansen remembered him as a "romantic reporter, one to whom the meticulous accuracy of a steno-
graphic report was abominable and uninspired." Once Hecht
was covering an out-of-town hanging, and the editor wired
him to tone down the gruesome details in his story. Hecht

cheekily wired back, "Will try to make hanging as pleasant as possible."[87] He went to Germany for the News after the armistice in 1918 and incorporated the experience into Erik Dorn. In 1923, he started his own paper, the Chicago Literary Times, which he edited for two years.[88]

Hecht was hailed after the publication of Erik Dorn as one of the real hopes of American literature. Although he became well known for his plays and movie scripts--The Front Page (1928), written with his frequent collaborator Charles MacArthur, is a minor classic of both the stage and screen--he never fulfilled his initial promise. Frederick Dupree put it bluntly: Hecht had "more gross talent than net accomplishment."[89]

The sardonic humor that distinguishes The Front Page is nowhere evident in Erik Dorn. Rather, the novel grimly follows Dorn's futile attempts to overcome his spiritual inertia. A veteran editor on a Chicago paper, he displays a "perfect affinity toward his work." But it is mean and meaningless work, as he realizes behind his "automatic efficiency." The thought occurs to him that "if there's anything worthy the absurdity of life it's a newspaper--gibbering, whining, strutting, sprawled in attitudes of worship before the nine-and-ninety lies of the moment--a caricature of absurdity itself."[90]

Everything Dorn touches, he harms. His wife "had after seven years of marriage found herself drained, hollowed out as by some tenaciously devouring insect."[91] He deserts her for Rachel, a young artist. She, in turn, is sucked dry and discarded.

Dorn and his inamorata had run off to New York, where he took a job on the New Opinion. The magazine sends him to Europe to report on the postwar turmoil. While abroad, he writes a book about Germany that makes him famous. Not even fame, however, can fill his emptiness. "The rivers ... flow to the sea and life flows to death," he says. "And there is nothing else of consequence for intelligence to record."[92]

The plot takes a melodramatic twist right out of a grade-B movie when Dorn is attacked in a Munich café by George Hazlitt, his former rival for Rachel and now a lawyer with the American army of occupation. In their struggle, Hazlitt is shot and killed. Dorn returns to the United States a "wife deserter, a seducer, a murderer."[93]

Where other protagonists graduate from journalism, he drifts back to his old job in Chicago and living burial. The interest he used to feel in his work is gone and long past recovering:

> His world. It was the same, only now he was conscious of it. Before he had sat in its midst unaware of more than a detail here, a gesture there. Now he seemed to be looking down from an airplane --a strange bird's eye view of things unstrange.
> He returned to his desk. The scene again reached out to embrace him.... He felt its embrace and yet remained outside it. There were things in him now that could never be a part of the unchanging old shop.[94]

For Dorn, there are, as Kenneth Patchen wrote, "so many little dyings that it doesn't matter / which one of them is death."[95] The novel ends with him standing at a window in his apartment, watching night come. The snow-covered buildings in the dark look like a "skeleton world"--a counterpart to T. S. Eliot's The Waste Land and F. Scott Fitzgerald's "Valley of Ashes."[96] Dorn is a casualty of his country and his day and the empty newspaper game.

From 1890 to 1930, fiction portrayed journalism in highly contradictory terms. Journalism invited college men into its ranks; it knocked the college clean out of them. Journalism nurtured aspiring young writers; it destroyed their talent. Journalism was a school of practical experience; it was a cemetery crowded with graves and ghosts.

The split image reflected the ambivalence of reporters-turned-novelists who got out of journalism but never totally escaped its pull. To feed their fiction, they cannibalized incidents, characters, and attitudes from their newspaper careers. They echoed the cynical talk of the city room on slow-news nights. And, by a curious mental alchemy, they transformed into their very own the savage criticisms flung at the press by the custodians of official culture. They left journalism divided within themselves about what it did

for them and to them. Memory spoke in hot type that caut-
erized the wounds in their minds.

References

1. Joseph A. Altsheler, Gutherie of the Times (New
York: Doubleday, Page, 1904), p. 54.
2. Joseph Pulitzer, "The College of Journalism,"
North American Review, May 1904, p. 642.
3. F. M. Colby, "Attacking the Newspapers," Bookman, Vol. XV, Aug. 1902, p. 534.
4. Thomas Griffith, The Waist-High Culture (New
York: Harper & Brothers, 1959), p. 65.
5. Norman Hapgood, The Changing Years (New
York: Farrar & Rinehart, 1930), p. 122.
6. Samuel G. Blythe, The Making of a Newspaper
Man (Philadelphia: Henry Altemus, 1912; reprint ed., Westport, Conn.: Greenwood Press, 1970), pp. 217-18.
7. Quoted in Stanley Walker, City Editor (New
York: Frederick A. Stokes, 1934), pp. 4-5.
8. Shuman, Practical Journalism, pp. 25, 46, 56.
9. Julius Chambers, News Hunting on Three Continents (New York: Mitchell Kennerley, 1921), p. 308.
10. Richard O'Connor, The Scandalous Mr. Bennett
(New York: Doubleday, 1962), pp. 77, 166-67.
11. Ibid., p. 78.
12. George Britt, Forty Years--Forty Millions: The
Career of Frank A. Munsey (New York: Farrar & Rinehart,
1935), pp. 111, 115.
13. Quoted in Britt, Forty Years, p. 248.
14. Ibid., p. 244.
15. Whitelaw Reid, "Recent Changes in the Press,"
American and English Studies, Vol. 2 (London: Smith,
Elder, 1914), p. 309.
16. George Juergens, Joseph Pulitzer and the New
York World (Princeton: Princeton University Press, 1966),
pp. 238-39.
17. Quoted in Commager, American Mind, p. 53.
18. Quoted in Simon Michael Bessie, Jazz Journalism
(New York: Dutton, 1938; reprint ed., Russel & Russel,
1969), p. 40.
19. Quoted in Juergens, Joseph Pulitzer, pp. 110-11.
20. Quoted in Juergens, Joseph Pulitzer, p. 34.
21. Finley Peter Dunne, Observations by Mr. Dooley
(New York: Harper & Brothers, 1902), p. 240.

22. Quoted in Commager, American Mind, p. 69.

23. Quoted in Schudson, Discovering the News, p. 114.

24. Ibid., footnote 57, p. 208.

25. Quoted in Tebbel, The Life and Good Times of William Randolph Hearst, p. 79.

26. "Our Chamber of Horrors," Outlook, Sept. 30, 1911, p. 261.

27. Quoted in Bessie, Jazz Journalism, p. 19.

28. Theodore Dreiser, "Out of My Newspaper Days," Bookman, Vol. LIV, Sept. 1921-Feb. 1922, p. 429.

29. Richard Harding Davis, "The Reporter Who Made Himself King," The King's Jackal (New York: Scribner's, 1904), p. 143. The story originally appeared in McClure's Magazine in 1891.

30. Walker, City Editor, p. 41.

31. Robert C. Bannister, Jr., Ray Stannard Baker (New Haven: Yale University Press, 1966), pp. ix, 39-40, 67-68.

32. Ray Stannard Baker, "Pippins," Youth's Companion, Sept. 7, 1899, p. 435.

33. Ibid.

34. Ibid., pp. 435-36.

35. Quoted in Sutton, Education for Journalism, p. 9.

36. Quoted in Charles J. Rosebault, When Dana Was The Sun (New York: Robert M. McBride, 1931; reprint ed., Westport, Conn.: Greenwood Press, 1970), p. 289.

37. Davis, "Reporter Who Made Himself King," pp. 142-43.

38. Wayland Wells Williams, Goshen Street (New York: Frederick A. Stokes, 1920), pp. 88-89.

39. Edward Hungerford, The Copy Shop (New York: Putnam's, 1925), p. 32.

40. Will Irwin, The Making of a Reporter (New York: Putnam's, 1942), p. 109.

41. Williams, Stolen Story, pp. 68-70.

42. Ibid., pp. 76, 87, 93, 96.

43. Dreiser, "Out of My Newspaper Days," p. 210.

44. Ibid., p. 428.

45. Theodore Dreiser, Free and Other Stories (New York: Boni & Liveright, 1918), pp. 163, 166, 199-200.

46. Ibid., p. 76.

47. Ibid., pp. 77, 100-101.

48. Ibid., pp. 110-111.

49. Ibid., p. 111.

50. Hughes, News and the Human Interest Story, p. 97.

51. Stanley J. Kunitz and Howard Haycraft, Twentieth Century Authors (New York: H. W. Wilson, 1942), pp. 631-32.

52. Ibid., pp. 818-19.

53. Meyer Levin, Reporter (New York: John Day, 1929), p. 128.

54. Ibid., p. 35.

55. Ibid., p. 267.

56. Phillips, Great God Success, p. 11.

57. Davis, "Reporter Who Made Himself King," pp. 142-43.

58. Jesse Lynch Williams, Stolen Story, p. 96.

59. Ben Ames Williams, Splendor (New York: Dutton, 1927), p. 205.

60. Malcolm H. Ross, Penny Dreadful (New York: Coward-McCann, 1929), p. 57.

61. Gene Fowler, Trumpet in the Dust (New York: Liveright, 1930), p. 294.

62. Shuman, Practical Journalism, pp. 148, 151.

63. Brander Matthews, "An Interview with Miss Marlenspuyk," Outlines in Local Color (New York: Scribner's, 1921), p. 170.

64. Elizabeth G. Jordan, "Miss Van Dyke's Best Story," Tales of the City Room (New York: Scribner's, 1898), p. 228.

65. Kunitz and Haycraft, Twentieth Century Authors, pp. 444-45.

66. Ferber, Dawn O'Hara, p. 47.

67. Ibid., pp. 49-50.

68. Ibid., pp. 99-100.

69. Williams, Stolen Story, pp. 220, 256, 270.

70. For a detailed account of the clash over realism in the 1890s, see Grant C. Knight, The Critical Period in American Literature (Chapel Hill: University of North Carolina Press, 1951). Also of interest--and amusement-- is Thomas Beer, The Mauve Decade (Garden City, N.Y.: Garden City Publishing, 1926).

71. Alden Whitman, afterword to Stephen French Whitman's Predestined, pp. 465, 473-74.

72. Whitman, Predestined, p. 56.

73. Ibid., pp. 56-57.

74. Ibid., pp. 63, 117, 153.

75. Ibid., p. 253. Gene Fowler characterized the

copy desk as a graveyard for journalistic gunfighters who were slow on the draw in Skyline (New York: Viking, 1961), pp. 225-26.

76. Whitman, Predestined, p. 357.

77. Ibid., p. 382.

78. Frederick Lewis Allen, Only Yesterday (New York: Harper & Brothers, 1931; paperback ed., New York: Harper & Row, 1964), p. 238.

79. Quoted in Allen, Only Yesterday, p. 116.

80. John O. Lyons, in studying the development of another literary genre, found that the "real distinction between the novels which came before and those which came after the war is their depiction of social, and specifically sexual, behavior." The College Novel in America (Carbondale, Ill.: Southern Illinois University Press, 1962), p. 24.

81. Fowler, Trumpet in the Dust, p. 353.

82. Edwin Emery and Michael Emery, The Press and America: An Interpretive History of the Mass Media, 5th ed. (Englewood Cliffs, N.J.: Prentice-Hall, 1984), p. 389.

83. Bent, Ballyhoo, p. 41.

84. Quoted in Bessie, Jazz Journalism, p. 19.

85. Bent, Ballyhoo, p. 196.

86. Ben Hecht, Gaily, Gaily (New York: New American Library, 1963), p. 207.

87. Quoted in Harry Hansen, Midwest Portraits (New York: Harcourt, Brace, 1923), pp. 327-28.

88. Kunitz and Haycraft, Twentieth Century Authors, pp. 631-32.

89. Quoted in Kunitz and Haycraft, Twentieth Century Authors, p. 632.

90. Hecht, Erik Dorn, pp. 18-19.

91. Ibid., p. 12.

92. Ibid., p. 344.

93. Ibid., p. 376.

94. Ibid., p. 391.

95. Kenneth Patchen, "And What with the Blunders," The Love Poems of Kenneth Patchen (San Francisco: City Lights Books, 1972), p. 23.

96. Hecht, Erik Dorn, p. 409.

Chapter III

## THE CRUSADER WITH A BROKEN LANCE

What the mob thirsts for is not good government in itself, but the merry chase of a
definite exponent of bad government.
> --H. L. Mencken, "Newspaper
> Morals"

"A sustaining myth of journalism," press critic Edward Jay
Epstein has said, "holds that every great government scandal is revealed through the work of enterprising reporters
who by one means or another pierce the official veil of secrecy."[1] The newspaper fiction published from 1890 to 1930
reflects that myth and, in fact, may have been partly responsible for creating it.

Quite a few novels and short stories feature a crusading journalist. The crusader often arrives in town a stranger. Perhaps he has inherited a struggling newspaper from
a distant relative, perhaps he has drifted onto the scene in
search of a job. In either instance, he finds a community
controlled by greedy businessmen or corrupt politicians or
machine gun-toting gangsters. Acting as an extralegal
force, he routs the evildoers. He is a messianic figure who
materializes out of nowhere to break the midnight conspiracies that rule the sunlit streets and to protect the innocent
and defenseless from the depraved and strong.

The story pattern usually ends in one of two ways.
Sometimes the crusader is rewarded with the love of a

beautiful woman, fame and prosperity for his paper, and promotion out of daily journalism. He becomes a leader in the community he helped save. His leadership may be formally recognized by election to political office, as happens to John Harkless in Booth Tarkington's The Gentleman from Indiana, Billy Gutherie in Joseph A. Altsheler's Gutherie of the Times, Jeremy Robson in Samuel Hopkins Adams's Common Cause, and Sabra Cravat in Edna Ferber's Cimarron.

Other times, the crusader disappears as mysteriously as he appeared. Such is the case in Olin L. Lyman's Micky (1905) and Louis Dodge's Whispers (1920). The crusader establishes the basis for civilization in what had been a moral wilderness, only to vanish once his utility is gone. He resembles the cowboy hero who sets the stage for frontier settlement and his own demise by driving off Indians and gunning down outlaws. Yancey Cravat, Sabra's husband in Cimarron, more than resembles a cowboy; he is one. Conspicuously attired in high-heeled Texas-star boots, a pair of fancy revolvers, and a white sombrero, the founding editor of the Oklahoma Wigwam is "famed as the deadliest shot in all the deadly shooting Southwest."[2]

As in a double exposure, the image of journalism as a cemetery hazily emerges in many novels behind the image of it as a crusade, and complicates the picture. The protagonist of Micky, a tramp newspaperman whose fearless reporting smashes the political machine in an unidentified Eastern city, cautions a cub:

> You'll find this "career," as you call it, is a good deal like a hobby horse. Pleasant motion, but doesn't land you anywhere. There's nothing to it. I heard you talking the other day about "the great equipment it gives a fellow for a start in life." That's all right if taken in time, like the measles, but let me tell you something. You stick to this, and stick and stick, and by the time you're ready for that start, you'll be backin' up.[3]

The crusader graduates to politics or fades into the faceless night. Even when journalism is a cure for social ills, it exhibits vicious side effects for those foolish enough to try to make a career of it.

Further complicating things is the notion expressed in several works that the crusader is perpetrating a cruel hoax. He merely pretends to fight for equality and justice in order to blind the public to his true purpose. Howard, the publisher of the New York News-Record in David Graham Phillips's The Great God Success, quietly drops a crusade against the "Coal Conspiracy" when he is shown it will jeopardize his investments, and he accepts the bribe of an ambassadorship in exchange for his paper's support of the plutocracy's presidential candidate. In Miriam Michelson's A Yellow Journalist (1905), the owner of the San Francisco News, Offield, has a secret $40,000-a-year contract with the political boss of California to refrain from attacking a power company in print. Journalism is no cleaner, and perhaps a lot dirtier, than the vermin it is supposed to stamp out. "I swear to you my wrist is tired of signing checks for Offield and his like," the boss complains to Michelson's heroine.

> Look! here is a new demand from a Southern paper --it needs new presses. And here is a Northern one that wants a linotype machine. And here in the city is one that must have a color press.... A graceless herd of traitors they are, these newspaper proprietors who shamelessly put themselves up for sale; who pull at your coat and smirkingly try to catch your eye and force their venality upon your attention, yet who will not stay bought....[4]

David Holman, the Hearst-like publisher in William Richard Hereford's The Demagog (1909), is another false messiah. He editorially condemns machine politicians and the rich while secretly plotting with both to steal his party's presidential nomination. Utterly devoid of conscience, he would take the strength of the "great formless mass of the people ... [and] exploit it for his own ends as, in an earlier day, the traders from Africa exploited the strength of the slaves they captured."[5]

In presenting these sinister characters, fiction was responding to the growth of newspaper monopolies. There were eight chains in 1900, and they controlled twenty-seven papers and about ten percent of daily circulation. By the close of the decade, there were a dozen chains, and the number of papers under their control had doubled.[6] As concentration of ownership increased, so did anxiety that a few ruthless publishers would use their exclusive power over the national mind to rule--or, rather, misrule--the country.

For the twentieth-century newspaper, the "paramount object is to make money," Edwin L. Shuman said. "If a publisher sees that a sensational style sells the most papers, he is strongly tempted to give the public a 'yellow journal,' just as a merchant gives his customers calico if they want it instead of silk."[7] Like big pictures and titillating stories of sex, crime, and violence, crusading was a special attraction of yellow journalism. The New York Press repeatedly assailed bribery in city government, and the Philadelphia North American exposed local bossism and food adulteration. In 1901, the St. Louis Post-Dispatch defeated a gang of political grafters when it persuaded one of them to turn state's evidence.[8] Newspapers, Rollo Ogden wrote in Atlantic Monthly in 1906, make "every headline an officer ... an advance section of the Day of Judgment."[9] The cries for reform echoing through the popular press unnerved the supporters of the status quo. Their fear of rising democracy also colored the portrait of the crusader as a sham or charlatan.

From 1890 to 1920, America was transformed by industrialization, urbanization, and immigration. The great potential wealth of the country dazzled the mind. Capital, labor, natural resources, and inventiveness were in plentiful supply. Life was getting better, and Americans had high expectations for themselves and their children.

But the transformation of America into a complex modern society produced bewildering and painful contradictions. Poverty stood out starkly in an era of unparalleled prosperity. Municipal corruption was intolerable at a time when the city was hailed as a center of civilization.[10] Anger and frustration over such disparities gave birth to the Progressive movement, which lasted roughly from the Spanish-American War to the First World War. One historian has dubbed Progressivism the "Revolt of the American Conscience."[11] Progressives wanted to open up government, regulate business, and help the underdog.

The press joined the fight for reform out of a mixture

of motives. It benefited from anything that caused a stir and attracted readers, and so, pitched in. Some journalists, however, were genuinely outraged by the social problems they saw everywhere. The indignation that animated the Progressive Era can be glimpsed in the titles of some contemporary magazine articles: "The Shame of the Cities," "The Treason of the Senate," "Frenzied Finance," and "The Great American Fraud." William Allen White, publisher-editor of the Emporia (Kan.) Gazette and a leading Progressive, said, "Newspapers, magazines, books--every representative outlet for public opinion was turned definitely away from the scoundrels who had in the last third or quarter of the old century cast themselves in monumental brass as heroes. The muckrakers were melting it down."[12]

Newspaper fiction was quick to incorporate the muckraker into its regular cast of characters. Crusades of all kinds are conducted in its pages: John Harkless battles vigilantes in Booth Tarkington's The Gentleman from Indiana (1899); Billy Woods kicks the boodlers out of city hall in Jesse Lynch Williams's The Day-Dreamer (1906); Lawrence Ashmore thwarts a ring of stock-market manipulators in Charles Agnew MacLean's The Mainspring (1912); Hal Surtaine exposes patent-medicine fakers in Samuel Hopkins Adams's The Clarion (1914).

The crusaders who are rewarded with political office for their efforts are close relations of the protagonist of the Progressive novel, which Henry F. May called "one of the simplest literary genres that ever existed." As May describes the basic plot, a "young lawyer, usually of sound family, went into politics to help the people. Suddenly, perhaps when he was offered a bribe, he realized that there was a system. Challenging the powerful and sinister bosses, he fought relentlessly until, in a final climactic scene with crowds cheering and the heroine waiting just off stage with brimming eyes, the bosses went down to defeat."[13] Substitute the word journalist for lawyer, and the result is a pretty fair description of The Gentleman from Indiana or Gutherie of the Times.

Despite the highly publicized problems of poverty, political corruption, crime, and concentrated wealth, the period between the Spanish-American War and the First World War has been characterized as "The Good Years."[14]

"It is doubtful whether the people of the United States have ever been more cheerful, more self-assured, more light-hearted...," literary historian Grant C. Knight said of the first decade of the twentieth century, "and this in the face of present and foreseen dangers." For all the reform-minded literature that clamored to be read, historical romances and Graustarkian fiction dominated the best-seller lists between 1901 and 1910.[15]

Samuel Hopkins Adams, David Graham Phillips, Ray Stannard Baker, and Samuel Merwin had muckraked for magazines, but the sentimentality of the feminine reading public seems to have inhibited former muckrakers from crusading in their newspaper novels. Only Adams in The Clarion and Phillips in The Great God Success significantly drew on the knowledge of politics, business, and finance they had gained as reporters.[16] The others cut their writings to fit current fashion and offered a strongly perfumed version of life. Reform ended for them in the banality of popular literature.

Progressivism itself was a casualty of the First World War. After government blindness and bungling had caused the butchery of millions on the battlefields of Europe, it was difficult to believe that government rules and regulations could create a just society at home. Moreover, the long nightmare of the trenches shattered the traditional equation of history with progress, the meliorist vision of humanity proudly marching out of the darkness toward the light.[17] The struggle to make the world safe for democracy had exhausted the country's capacity to sacrifice for ideals. Americans needed to convalesce from the fever and delirium of the war effort.

Throughout the twenties, the crusading journalist was still a standard character in fiction, but he lacked the zeal of his predecessors. "[N]ow and then when I stumble on a fact which is news, I print it," says Arthur Morton, the protagonist of John C. Mellett's Ink (1930) and an example of the amoral crusader of the Jazz Age. "If readers are surprised, or horrified, or startled into action, that is all right with me. If not, all right too. I'm only interested in printing things that will interest them...."[18]

Prohibition, which was in effect from 1920 to 1933,

hatched a whole new brood of dragons for such reluctant crusaders as Morton to slay. Frederick Lewis Allen observed, "There have always been gangs and gangsters in American life and doubtless always will be; there has always been corruption of city officials and doubtless always will be; yet it is ironically true, none the less, that the outburst of corruption and crime ... in the nineteen-twenties was immediately occasioned by the attempt to banish the temptations of liquor from the American home."[19] Gangsters seemed to be everywhere, except in jail. They gave orders to judges and prosecutors, entertained politicians at banquets, slaughtered each other in bloody wars, and were buried in $10,000 caskets at gaudy funerals.[20]

"Gangland's one-way rides, shoot-outs, and bombings were big news in the Prohibition days," recalled William T. Moore, a rewrite man on the old Chicago Herald & Examiner. A crime reporter was expected to pal around with underworld figures to keep track of what they were doing. And gangsters, Moore said, "had a curious affinity to newspaper folk...." Chicago Tribune reporter Fred Pasley, who wrote the first biography of Al Capone, was a welcome guest at Capone's parties.[21]

From front-page headlines to newspaper fiction was a short leap. While machine guns rattled from the windows of speeding automobiles, authors rattled out an accompaniment on their typewriters. They turned loose an army of hard-boiled newspapermen to do battle with bootleggers and grafters.

Crime news had become a staple of journalism decades before Prohibition, and the detective-reporters of the yellow press provided another model for the fictional crusader. Isaac D. White was a celebrated member of the crime-busting fraternity. His most brilliant exploit involved an unknown man who entered the New York offices of Russell Sage and hurled a bomb at the financier. The bomb exploded prematurely, blowing the hurler to bits and killing a clerk. Thousands of police worked for days to identify the would-be assassin, but finally they gave up.

Meanwhile, White obtained a button and a patch of cloth from the bomb-thrower's suit. The button was made by a Boston firm whose name was stamped on it. White took it to the manufacturers, and they gave him a list of the clothiers in New York they had supplied with buttons of that type. He checked the haberdashers and tailors until he found the one who had made the suit of which the patch of cloth was a sample. The tailor had the man's name and address, and White had his scoop.[22]

Detective-reporters were so visible and annoying that Kansas editors, meeting in solemn conclave in 1910, approved a code of ethics containing the following provision: "We condemn against justice the practice of reporters making detectives and spies of themselves in their endeavors to investigate the guilt or innocence of those under suspicion."[23] But in 1927, Silas Bent lamented the passing of White and his kind. Not only had they brought a certain picturesqueness to journalism, they also had served an important function. "When we compare," Bent said, "the long list of mysteries solved by the press in the latter part of the century and the early part of this with the long list of murder mysteries since then which remain mysteries, we begin to suspect that the amateur detective-reporter had his uses."[24]

Melville Stone, founder of the Chicago Daily News, was not above playing detective, and he once chased an absconding bank president halfway round the world. Stone explained that the "exposure of crime and the punishment of criminals were of great value to the community and gratifying to the business office, because they created sensations, made us notable, enlarged our circulation, and filled our coffers."[25] It was a desire for exclusive news more than a passion for justice that inspired detective-reporters to feats of ingenuity. The scoop was, in Will Irwin's words, the "royal road to prestige, circulation, and prosperity," and city rooms "lived in a state of murderous competition."[26]

The mania to be the fastest to gather the news and the first to report it is enshrined in fiction. After solving a case that had baffled the authorities, Ben Crisp, the sleuth in Irvin S. Cobb's Alias Ben Alibi (1925), says: "I'm not concerned about the ends of justice. I wanted to show up Mr. Police Commissioner Dudley and likewise Mr. District Attorney Salmon.... And, most of all, I wanted to put the Star across for the biggest beat in years...."[27]

There are virtually no limits to what fictional journalists

will do to run down their quarry and score a scoop. "[A] reporter," Crisp declares, "is justified in almost any course short of murder that will help him get at the inside story-- the one that's covered up."[28] In Olin L. Lyman's Micky, a tramp newspaperman chloroforms a political boss and, while the man lies unconscious on the floor, takes incriminating documents from his coat pocket. Rhoda Massey of Miriam Michelson's A Yellow Journalist bribes, cheats, steals, and generally acts like a thug. Her managing editor is blithely indifferent to her criminal methods of reporting. "A newspaper is a business property, not a school of ethics," he remarks. "All that the office knows of Miss Massey's manner of doing things is that she never fails."[29]

Often justice is merely an incidental outcome of the relentless search for exclusive news. The journalist, as the title of a 1920 novel by Sydney Williams puts it, is An Unconscious Crusader. Michelson's sob sister has selfish motives and resorts to dishonest tactics, but she uncovers political graft all the same.

Of course, some protagonists do possess a wide-awake social conscience. John Harkless in Booth Tarkington's The Gentleman from Indiana intentionally sets out to right the world's wrongs. Tarkington began the novel in 1893, a few months after he graduated from Princeton.[30] The writing of the early chapters went smoothly, but then the narrative abruptly bogged down. "It wouldn't budge," Tarkington recalled. "The hero stuck fast in the middle of a walk he was taking--he wouldn't take another step." The novel remained unfinished for five years.

Viola Roseboro, a manuscript reader for McClure's, has been credited with "discovering" Tarkington. She strode into the office one morning with tears in her eyes, exclaiming, "Here is a serial sent by God Almighty for McClure's Magazine!" She was holding a copy of The Gentleman from Indiana. S. S. McClure asked Hamlin Garland for a second opinion, and Garland wrote to Tarkington: "Mr. McClure has given me your manuscript. You are a novelist."

After the manuscript was accepted, Tarkington visited McClure at the magazine's office in New York. "You," the publisher said, grasping the young writer's hand, "you are to be the greatest of the new generation, and we will help you to be!" The Gentleman from Indiana was serialized in abridged form in McClure's in 1899. Publication of a story by Anthony Hope, author of the best-selling Prisoner of Zenda, was postponed to make room for it. Reading the novel today, however, it is difficult to understand what all the fuss was about.

Having attended an Eastern college and worked for some years on a New York newspaper, Harkless returns to his native Indiana a stranger. He has used his savings to buy a moribund weekly, the Carlow County Herald in Platville. "I wanted to run a paper myself," he explains, "and to build a power!" He wields the Herald as if it were a flaming sword, smashing a ring of political grafters, exposing confidence men, and sending members of a vigilante group, the White Caps, to prison. He intercedes for truth and justice whenever the authorities prove "either lackadaisical or timorous."[31]

Harkless is also a reformer on a more personal level. Soon after arriving in Platville, he hires Old Fisbee, the town drunk, as a reporter. Fisbee is transformed almost overnight into a responsible citizen. It is one of the few instances in fiction where journalism rejuvenates, rather than wrecks, a character.

Notwithstanding the success of his paper, Harkless is a melancholy young man. He believes he has let down his college chums, who called him the Great Harkless and thought he would be "minister to England in a few years." Platville is a long way from the Court of St. James's. Harkless feels he has "dropped out of the world."[32] His depression is deepened by his frustrated love for beautiful Helen Sherwood. Unknown to Harkless, she is Old Fisbee's daughter, given up for adoption as a little girl after her mother died. Much of the plot turns--and very slowly at that--on the creaky device of mistaken identity.

When Harkless is beaten and shot by the White Caps in retaliation for his crusade against them, Helen Sherwood (or Fisbee) takes charge of the Herald. She is the literary counterpart of the Gibson Girl, the Christy Girl, the Gilbert Girl, a "parade of incredibly handsome, smartly dressed young things" who sprang from the pens of illustrators in the 1890s.[33] These mythical creatures graced calendars, magazine covers, and the lids of candy boxes, and they flattered vain women with an improved portrait of themselves.

The Tarkington Girl has no journalistic training, yet she ably runs the paper during Harkless's convalescence. In fact, she remakes the weekly into a daily, Platville into an oil boomtown, and Harkless into a congressman. And she does it all in an oh-so-ladylike manner. She even worries that the reporters, who have no rubbers or umbrellas, will catch colds going out in the rain after news.

Eventually, the confusion over Helen Fisbee's (or Sherwood's) identity is cleared up, and she and Harkless swear eternal love and head for Washington, D.C. Tarkington himself won a seat as a Republican in the Indiana legislature of 1903. Both he and his hero were products of the special spirit of the Progressive Era. "It was a period dominated almost exclusively ... by the passion for reform," Alfred Kazin observed. "A generation arose determined to mold its destiny by politics...."[34]

What will happen to the Herald while Harkless is off pursuing a political career is left hanging. Perhaps this was inevitable. Unlike most authors of newspaper fiction, Tarkington never toiled in daily journalism, though he did take a course in reporting at Purdue University in 1890.[35] The result is a newspaper novel largely lacking in authentic detail--the smell of printer's ink, the rumble of the presses.

Ray Stannard Baker still considered The Gentleman from Indiana "one of the biggest stories of the decade."[36] Theodore Roosevelt, on the other hand, was disgusted by its "realism."[37] Early installments in McClure's also provoked protests from some country editors who prematurely concluded that Tarkington was arraigning small-town America and painting his home state in too somber colors. With a surer estimate of his art, the public reached for the novel when it was published in book form to enjoy the sentimental romance of its idealized hero and heroine. The Gentleman from Indiana made the monthly best-seller lists twice in 1900 and continued in demand for years. It was reprinted more than a dozen times, translated into at least six languages, produced as a movie, and excerpted for anthologies.[38]

Although the novel was a financial bonanza for Tarkington, he came to view it as an artistic failure. In later writings, he moved away from its saccharine style and excessive plotting, and received Pulitzer Prizes for The Magnificent Ambersons (1918) and Alice Adams (1921). Tarkington, like many others who wrote newspaper fiction, did his finest work outside the genre, which chiefly became the province of dilettantes and hacks.

A decade and a half after the appearance of The Gentleman from Indiana, fiction was still following the same basic pattern in portraying the crusading editor. The pattern is present at its sentimental worst in Samuel Hopkins Adams's The Clarion. Adams had gone to the New York Sun straight from college. Nine years of reporting were enough--"in fact, too much," he said--and he quit the paper to join the staff of McClure's. He subsequently shifted to another muckraking organ, Collier's. Will Irwin, a colleague there, described Adams as a "born muckraker" who "gloried in combat." In October 1905, the magazine began running Adams's "The Great American Fraud," an exposé of the $60-million-a-year patent-medicine industry. The series has been credited with furthering passage of the first Pure Food and Drug Act.[39]

Adams drew on his muckraking background in writing The Clarion. Its hero, Hal Surtaine, is the twenty-five-year-old son of an old quack who has made a bundle selling patent medicines. After college and a long stay in Europe, Hal returns to Worthington ignorant of the corruption underlying the family fortune. So when a local daily denounces his father's most popular nostrum, he is outraged and strikes back by buying the paper.

He immediately has cause for second thoughts. Ellis McGuire, an editor on the Clarion, charges that it is Hal's "kind that's made journalism the sewer of professions, full of the scum and drainings of every other trade's failures. What chance have we got to develop ideals when you outsiders control the whole business?" McGuire paints for him a glorious picture of what a newspaper might be: "A teacher and a preacher. A force to tear down and to build up. To rip this old town wide open and remould it nearer to the heart's desire!"[40]

Hal is converted by McGuire's "hot idealism." He determines to transform the Clarion into the "cleanest, decentest newspaper in the city." It is a bitter struggle. For years, "suppression and manipulation of the news" has characterized journalism in Worthington. When Hal begins to "give the news without fear or favor," the city fathers are mortified.[41] Libel suits are threatened, advertising is withdrawn. The paper totters on the brink of bankruptcy.

But Hal persists in his knight-errantry, to the point of exposing his father's patent-medicine business as "all lies! Lies and murders!" He also publishes the fact that the woman he loves owns one of the tenements where a typhoid epidemic is raging. Such things are hard on him; however, he can do no less, for news is "only a small name for Truth. Good men have died for that."[42]

Naturally, Hal triumphs in the end. Unable to ruin his paper, business leaders decide to take advantage of its large circulation and advertise in it. His father, who had held that "hifalutin notions" about a newspaper being a "palladium and the voice of the people" was a lot of "guff," changes his mind and stops manufacturing patent medicines. And Hal's girl razes her tenement as a "confession" that he was right to criticize her.[43] As if all this were not enough, the President of the United States commends the Clarion for its part in eradicating the epidemic.

That Adams, an accomplished muckraker, shaped The Clarion to the established story pattern illustrates the crushing weight of literary stereotypes or the continual yearning of Americans for a messiah--or both. Readers found in the image of the crusading journalist something they could not find in life: a hero equal to their doubts and fears. Hal and his kind offered reassurance that the press was fighting on the side of the little guy and that simple and painless solutions existed for difficult and painful problems.

Adams wrote two more novels about newspaper crusaders, Common Cause (1919) and Success (1921). Common Cause is a replay of The Clarion, except instead of battling patent-medicine quackery, editor Jeremy Robson battles pro-German sentiment in the mythical Midwestern state of Centralia during World War I. He is rewarded with love, prosperity and election to the U.S. Senate.

Success is a better, and bleaker, book. Errol Ban-
neker rises from stationmaster in a desert town in California
to editor of a yellow journal in New York. Along the way,
he compromises his principles, so that he finally reckons,
"If ever there was a word coined in hell, [it was] success."
He quits the paper and returns to the desert to pay penance
for his journalistic sins and--what else--write fiction. The
central theme of the novel is summed up by another character, veteran reporter Pop Edmonds, when he wonders whether
the "newspaper game isn't just too strong for us who try to
play it."[44]

The sudden clouding of Adams's vision of journalism
is a revealing development. As traditional American values
and beliefs were challenged by youths, women, intellectuals,
scientists, and bootleggers after World War I, newspaper fiction grew disillusioned with reform and pessimistic about the
future. The crusader of the twenties rode to the rescue on
a bony nag and armed with a broken lance.

It probably could have been predicted that he would
lose his enthusiasm for crusading. Fiction had always been
suspicious of the nature and role of the press. There was
the portrayal of journalism as either a school or a cemetery.
There were the false prophets of newsprint, Howard in
David Graham Phillips's The Great God Success and David
Holman in William Richard Hereford's The Demagog. Even
the honest crusader, the most positive of the literary images
of the journalist, had long had chinks in his armor.

In Joseph A. Altsheler's Gutherie of the Times, reporter Billy Gutherie exposes political corruption, clears the
wrongly accused, and still feels frustrated and restless. He
realizes that "he was in a way a maker of reputations for
many, but not for himself. Others, and it was he who made
it possible, were having their triumphs, but he remained the
same."[45] Michael O'Byrn, the "tattered knight of the road"
in Olin L. Lyman's Micky, calls journalism "this rotten business" and admits to sticking to it only because "I can't do
anything else."[46] These tiny seeds of disillusionment,
warmed by a black sun, burst into full bloom in postwar
fiction.

High Ground (1928) by Jonathan Brooks is a depressing portrait of a crusading journalist. "Jonathan Brooks"

was the pseudonym of John C. Mellett. His brother, Don, was editor of the Canton (Ohio) News. On July 16, 1926, Don Mellett was shot to death in a doorway by gangsters whose grip on local government the News was trying to break. The paper won the Pulitzer Prize for public service for its efforts.[47] But what set the tone of the novel was the assassination, not the award.

James Andrew Marvin publishes and edits the Daily Monitor in the small city of Summit, Illinois. His life story is related by his five children in separate chapters. While Mellett's use of point of view is sophisticated, his character- ization of Marvin is simplistic. As physically impressive as Yancey Cravat in Edna Ferber's Cimarron and as morally courageous as John Harkless in Booth Tarkington's The Gentleman from Indiana, he possesses a clearer notion of the journalist's mission than either. "A newspaper man," Marvin says, "should be like a judge. He should sit apart from contacts that might affect or influence his judgment. This is hard to do and still get the news; but it is neces- sary...." He takes the "high ground that a newspaper is an agency for good, for right, and for decency."[48]

A darker side of journalism is represented by the rival paper in town, the Tribune. Its editor, appropriately named Wolfe, conspires with corrupt politicians to ruin the Monitor. The sharp division of the press into good and evil papers that battle for the souls of readers is common in fiction. For example, the noble Day duels with the ignoble Earth in Jesse Lynch Williams's The Day-Dreamer, and the responsibile Vidette clashes with the irresponsible News in Louis Dodge's Whispers.

Also common is naming the owners and editors of the scandal sheets after animals and fish, as if journalism were the wild kingdom. The rich, arrogant publisher in Stephen Crane's Active Service is named Sturgeon. Beakman, who runs the News in Dodge's Whispers, is every bit as awful as his vulturous name implies. He delights in the "brow- beating of the friendless, the exposure of the weak, the thwarting of the ambitious."[49] Sturgeon, Beakman, and Wolfe are forerunners of perhaps the most personally vicious editor in all of fiction: Shrike in Nathanael West's Miss Lonelyhearts (1931). According to the unabridged edition of the Random House Dictionary, shrikes are birds with strong, hooked, and toothed bills that "impale their prey on thorns or suspend it from trees to tear it apart more easily, and are said to kill more than is necessary for them to eat."

Marvin fights Wolfe and the other carnivores in <u>High Ground</u> with "high-minded sledge-hammer type" editorials, but to no avail. He loses his paper to the bank, which in turn sells it to a national syndicate. With an "eye on dividends and earnings before anything else," the syndicate symbolizes the dangerous concentration of wealth and power that in earlier fiction was symbolized by the cruel, devious sultans of sensationalism.[50]

"The whole business of getting out a newspaper," Remsen Crawford observed in 1929, "has taken on such prodigious enlargement since the European war that little wonder can be felt at the growing trend for chain newspapers and the tendency to depend largely upon the big associations for a kind of Soviet system of news-gathering."[51] By 1927, there were fifty-five chains controlling 230 dailies with a combined circulation of 13 million.[52] It was feared in some quarters that the increasing standardization of the press would create an increasingly standardized society under more or less centralized direction. As Marvin explains:

> Summit <u>does</u> need a Summit newspaper. If we do
> not get it, we will before long become merely one of
> a chain of American cities, all alike, each noteworthy
> for nothing the others do not have, all working not
> for themselves, but for some other. We will become
> a city of plant managers, district superintendents,
> banking agents, employees all; as distinct from a
> city of owners ... and independent people....[53]

Mellett's novel ends apocalyptically, with Marvin dying in a fire that destroys the decrepit building that once housed the <u>Monitor</u>. The defeat and death of the old crusader demonstrate the futility of taking the high ground in a lowbred world. Marvin is burned at the stake, a martyr to freedom of the press, and out of the smoke and ashes rises a monstrous new age of corporate thuggery.

Because of the soaring costs of newsprint, machinery, and labor in the second decade of the twentieth century, a newspaper could no longer make money on circulation alone.

Advertising, and a lot of it, was necessary. Under these conditions, the business department began to carry greater influence. It seemed by the twenties that the economics of journalism had reduced the reporter to a chattel. He was only as honest as his employers and the employers of his employers, the advertisers, permitted. "[I]f his manager orders him to find a story where there is no story," John Macy wrote in 1922, "or to find a story of a certain kind where the facts lead to a story of another kind, he will not come back empty-handed lest he go away empty-handed on pay-day."[54] Five years later, H. L. Mencken remarked that while the journalist might think of himself as a professional, he remained a hired man. "His code of ethics are all right so long as they do not menace newspaper profits; the moment they do so the business manager, now quiescent, will begin to growl again."[55]

Scoop (1930), by two Providence, Rhode Island, newspapermen, James S. Hart and Garrett D. Byrnes, portrays journalism as a "prostitution" and the crusader as a pimp. Seumas "Snakes" Shiel, the protagonist, is a star reporter on a supposedly "respectable newspaper" in New England. The Evening Post proclaims under its masthead that it publishes "The Whole Truth and Nothing But the Truth." When a story might anger an advertiser, however, the business office hastily steps in. Snakes shrugs at the interference. "A newspaper," he cynically says, "is only people operating a machine."[56]

Yet Snakes differs from most fictional journalists in that he considers his cynicism a stigma rather than a badge of honor. In Whispers, Louis Dodge describes the staff of the News as a "class of men to whom the word cynicism was a delicious word. To be really cynical meant, to them, to be very superior. They greatly desired to be cynical, to be thought cynical."[57] By contrast, Snakes downs another whisky and gloomily reflects:

> Always newspapermen talked of work, method of handling the news, the city editor's women, the tendency of the pastor of the big downtown church toward young choir boys. Dirt, scandal, cynicism, belief in nothing but that the world is lousy with hypocrisy and married women who snickered at the backs of their husbands' necks at the thought of

> how easily they cheated them. Always the same,
> because they were always behind the scenes. Bet-
> ter to be simple and innocent and believe in good-
> ness and the triumph of virtue. Many great men
> had believed in it. Lack of capacity for belief was
> no sign of knowledge or genius.[58]

Newspaper crusaders in the fiction of the Progressive Era seldom doubted the justice of their cause. But the probings of science and the horrors of world war had robbed man of his nobility and certainty. Adrift in a relativistic universe where right and wrong are subjective, Snakes questions whether reform is even possible. "What the hell's the use of crusading against conditions," he asks, "when some other crusader will come along later, curse the condition which you imposed upon the world in order to get rid of the first one, and fight to impose a still newer condition?"[59] He nonetheless acts the part assigned him. His investigation into the sales of pardons to criminals topples the political boss of the state.

In the course of his crusade, Snakes meets and falls in love with the sister of a gangster. Their affair ends down the "road of great negation, privation, sadness, and death" when she is killed by a burst of machine-gun fire intended for her brother. Shattered by her murder and disgusted with journalism--a "parasitic business, this making a living recording blurbs and misfortune"--Snakes resigns from the Post and signs on a dirty old tramp steamer as a seaman. "I've got to go because I feel the horizon is the only place for me," he announces. "And that in spite of my mind which tells me there is no horizon. It's only the limit of my vision."[60]

Like much else in newspaper fiction from 1890 to 1930, crusading was portrayed ambiguously. On the one hand, it was an "occupation for the saint."[61] Crusaders seemed divinely inspired, leveling the fortresses of bootleggers with blasts of their trumpets, routing crooked officials with their flaming swords. As a pious old widow says to the battling heroine of Clarence B. Kelland's Contraband (1923), "Mebby He has marked you out and set you apart as His instrument."[62]

On the other hand, publishers of sensational journals

craved power and money, and crusading was merely a blind for their sordid ambitions. Or crusaders were driven by a desire for scoops, not a concern for justice. They exposed crime and corruption, but with criminal methods and from corrupt motives.

The cemetery was never far off. It formed a dark backdrop for the shining deeds of some of the sincerest crusaders. Accustomed to roving, they rarely remained in the communities they had released from evil spells. Instead, they were doomed to wander the earth, weary, ragged refugees of journalism. The protagonists of Olin L. Lyman's Micky and Louis Dodge's Whispers vanish into the night when their work is done. Yancey Cravat of Edna Ferber's Cimarron dies a shabby drifter in an accident in the Oklahoma oil fields.

By the 1920s, many crusaders were simply going through the motions. They had lost faith in the permanence of reform. "The boss is ditched," Snakes Shiel tells his editor, "and the Minority party will win the next election. The board of directors won't like that so much. But they needn't worry. They'll probably win the election after that."63 World War I marked the end of American innocence, and in the mad, whirling carnival of sex and cynicism that followed, the image of the crusading journalist shook and rattled and finally tumbled. The broken pieces glittered like the frozen tears of forsaken gods and forgotten heroes.

## References

1. Edward J. Epstein, Between Fact and Fiction: The Problem of Journalism (New York: Vintage Books, 1975), p. 19.
2. Edna Ferber, Cimarron (Greenwich, Conn.: Fawcett, 1971), p. 72.
3. Lyman, Micky, p. 134.
4. Miriam Michelson, A Yellow Journalist (New York: Appleton, 1905), p. 313.
5. William Richard Hereford, The Demagog (New York: Henry Holt, 1909), pp. 21-22.
6. Mott, American Journalism, p. 648.
7. Shuman, Practical Journalism, pp. 16-17.

8. Mott, American Journalism, p. 574.

9. Rollo Ogden, "Some Aspects of Journalism," The Profession of Journalism, p. 7.

10. Arthur Mann, ed., The Progressive Era, 2nd ed. (Hinsdale, Ill.: Dryden Press, 1975), p. 205.

11. Quoted in Mann, Progressive Era, p. 204.

12. William Allen White, The Autobiography of William Allen White (New York: Macmillan, 1946), p. 248.

13. Henry F. May, The End of American Innocence (New York: Knopf, 1959; reprint ed., Oxford: University Press, 1979), pp. 23-24.

14. Walter Lord, The Good Years (New York: Harper & Brothers, 1960).

15. For a detailed critique of American literary tastes in the first decade of the twentieth century, see Grant C. Knight, The Strenuous Age in American Literature (Chapel Hill: University of North Carolina, 1954).

16. Phillips's most recent biographer, Abe C. Ravitz, observed, "Fiction as an art, to Phillips, coincided with journalism...." David Graham Phillips, Twayne's United States Authors Series (New York: Twayne, 1966), p. 116.

17. Paul Fussell, The Great War and Modern Memory (London: Oxford University Press, 1975), p. 21.

18. John C. Mellett, Ink (Indianapolis: Bobbs-Merrill, 1930), p. 146.

19. Allen, Only Yesterday, pp. 219-20.

20. Henry Asbury, Gem of the Prairie: An Informal History of the Chicago Underworld (New York: Knopf, 1940), pp. 339-40.

21. William T. Moore, Dateline Chicago: A Veteran Newsman Recalls Its Heyday, with a foreword by Robert Cromie (New York: Taplinger, 1973), pp. 63, 167.

22. Remsen Crawford, "Aces of the Press," North American Review, Jan. 1929, p. 114.

23. Quoted in Walker, City Editor, p. 171.

24. Bent, Ballyhoo, p. 100.

25. Melville E. Stone, Fifty Years a Journalist (Garden City, N.Y.: Doubleday, Page, 1922), p. 179.

26. Irwin, Making of a Reporter, p. 52.

27. Irvin S. Cobb, Alias Ben Alibi (New York: George H. Doran, 1925), p. 57.

28. Ibid., p. 359.

29. Michelson, Yellow Journalist, p. 176.

30. The account of Tarkington's debut as a novelist is based on James Woodress, Booth Tarkington (Philadelphia:

Lippincott, 1954), pp. 61, 77; and Peter Lyon, Success Story: The Life and Times of S. S. McClure (New York: Scribner's, 1963), pp. 153-55.

31. Booth Tarkington, The Gentleman from Indiana (New York: Scribner's, 1915), pp. 68, 182.

An organization called the White Caps actually terrorized southern Indiana in the 1890s. The New York Sun sent star reporter Julian Ralph to investigate the situation. Recalling the assignment in his autobiography, Ralph described the vigilantes as "rascally, diseased, almost imbecile people" of the "poor white trash" order, and he said the region they infested "seemed to groan beneath a curse." He was shown the spot where half a dozen men and women returning from an open-air church had been ambushed. He also saw a house from which the White Caps had dragged two women, who were whipped because an "unjust suspicion had tarnished their names." Ralph, Making of a Journalist, p. 131.

32. Tarkington, Gentleman from Indiana, pp. 86, 183.
33. Beer, Mauve Decade, p. 58.
34. Alfred Kazin, "Three Pioneer Realists," Saturday Review of Literature, July 8, 1939, p. 3.
35. Woodress, Booth Tarkington, p. 53.
36. Bannister, Ray Stannard Baker, p. 67.
37. Commager, American Mind, p. 62.
38. Woodress, Booth Tarkington, pp. 81-84.
39. Kunitz and Haycraft, Twentieth Century Authors, p. 7; Irwin, Making of a Reporter, p. 155; Lyon, Success Story, pp. 246-50.
40. Samuel Hopkins Adams, The Clarion (New York: Grosset & Dunlap, 1914), p. 69.
41. Ibid., pp. 79, 96.
42. Ibid., pp. 341, 405.
43. Ibid., pp. 76, 408.
44. Samuel Hopkins Adams, Success (Boston: Houghton Mifflin, 1921), pp. 542, 546.
45. Altsheler, Gutherie of the Times, p. 236.
46. Lyman, Micky, pp. 29, 34, 136.
47. Mott, American Journalism, pp. 649-50.
48. John C. Mellett [Jonathan Brooks], High Ground (Indianapolis: Bobbs-Merrill, 1928), pp. 157, 305.
49. Louis Dodge, Whispers (New York: Scribner's, 1920), p. 13.
50. Mellett, High Ground, p. 288.
51. Crawford, "Aces of the Press," p. 110.

52. Allen, Only Yesterday, p. 189.

53. Mellett, High Ground, pp. 296-97.

54. John Macy, "Journalism," Civilization in the United States: An Inquiry by Thirty Americans, ed. by Harold E. Stearns (New York: Harcourt, Brace, 1922), pp. 39-40.

55. H. L. Mencken, "Journalism in America," A Gang of Pecksniffs, ed. by Theo Lippman, Jr. (New Rochelle, N.Y.: Arlingotn House, 1975), p. 130.

56. James S. Hart and Garrett D. Byrnes, Scoop (Boston: Little, Brown, 1930), pp. 10, 13, 103, 216.

57. Dodge, Whispers, p. 25.

58. Hart and Byrnes, Scoop, p. 13.

59. Ibid., pp. 15-16.

60. Ibid., pp. 216, 297, 303.

61. T. S. Eliot, "The Dry Salvages," Four Quartets (New York: Harcourt, Brace & World, 1943), p. 44.

62. Clarence Budington Kelland, Contraband (New York: A. L. Burt, 1923), p. 34.

63. Hart and Byrne, Scoop, p. 305.

Chapter IV

## THE SUNSHINE OF COUNTRY JOURNALISM

Another morning comes with its strange cure.
The earth is news.
                              --Wendell Berry, "The
                              Morning's News"

Most newspaper fiction published from 1890 to 1930 is set in
the city.[1] It was there, amid foul tenements and grimy factories, that the mass-circulation daily was born. Yellow
journalism was the unruly child of urbanization, industrialization, and immigration. The tens of thousands of people
who flocked to the city to find jobs in the wake of the Industrial Revolution swelled the size of the reading public.
They became the semiliterate patrons of the sensational
press.

The metropolis, pulsating at all hours with drama and
color, was the greatest arena for news. Fiction usually depicts the reporter scurrying from "one horizon of the city
to the other," gathering stories that will entertain or startle.
As a cub in Chicago, the hero of Henry Justin Smith's
Josslyn (1924) "traveled endlessly on street cars, and, like
a child, was happy, pressing his nose against a window-pane.
Many of the panoramas from car windows were bleak and
evil beyond words, but in the light of his eager interest
they blossomed."[2]

Inevitably, interest withers into premature cynicism,
and the feverish atmosphere of big-city dailies is largely

responsible. Driven by competition and thriving on sensationalism, metropolitan papers lay siege to the public with
scareheads and scoops. Somewhere over the rainbow of
popular literature, however, a more innocent kind of journalism flourishes. The country newspaper office provides
the setting for a handful of novels and short stories that
enshrine the virtues--or, more exactly, the virtuousness--
of small-town life. Nothing much happens in these works,
which is basically their point. Placidity is celebrated over
hustle, tradition over change. Country journals reflect and
reinforce the goodness of rural society.

"No article of faith was more passionately held" in
nineteenth-century America, Henry Steele Commager said,
"than that the farmer was the peculiarly beloved of God...."[3]
This belief was derived from the agrarianism of Jefferson's
time and the nature writings of the Romantic poets.[4] It
reappeared with renewed vigor in the 1840s, when a series
of melodramas was specifically created for touring companies
to perform in rural opera houses. According to Thomas
Beer, the stock characters in the plays included a "pure
farmer, a pure country girl, a villain from the city and an
urban adventuress." The moral was always the same: the
"country mice might have foibles or even stumble into sin
but their hearts were in the right place."[5]

In the last decade of the nineteenth century and the
first decade of the twentieth, an era of unprecedented urbanization, novels that idealized country folk achieved a
vogue, the most popular being Edward N. Westcott's David
Harum (1898). Such fiction answered the yearning of many
Americans for simpler, happier days. "For a few hours,"
literary historian James D. Hart observed, "the standardized
anonymity of New York, Chicago, and other metropolitan
centers could be put out of one's mind by reading about the
wholesome friendliness of small-town life."[6]

To an extent, then, authors were following literary
fashion in portraying country journalism as warm and sincere. But there was also a factual basis for the portrayal.
Country weeklies and small-town dailies eschewed yellow
techniques. "In these papers," Frank Luther Mott said,
"the gossip impulse was satisfied not by emphasis on crime
and scandal, but by the more kindly and matter-of-fact
record of social events, community enterprises, crops, visit-
ing, sickness, births, weddings, and deaths."[7]

Charles Moreau Harger explained in Atlantic Monthly in 1907 why the time had not yet arrived for the country newspaper to assume city airs: "The city journal is the paper of the masses; the country weekly or small daily is the paper of the neighborhood. One is general and impersonal; the other, direct and intimate. One is the marketplace; the other, the home. The distinction is not soon to be wiped out."[8] It survived even the rise of the tabloid press, whose rowdiness and sensationalism mirrored the new moral code of the Jazz Age. In 1932, the editor of the Mineville Mail, a Western weekly with a circulation of 1,105, told sociologist Albert Blumenthal: "If I printed the really interesting news in this town I would be run out of town. It would be a snap to put out the paper if I could put in scandal news but that stuff doesn't go in a small-town paper."[9]

The playing up of tragedy, crime, sex, and violence by metropolitan dailies was believed to cause a "ruinous, one-sided development" in newspapermen.[10]  By contrast, country journalism was thought to lead to a well-ripened personality.  Each June, college graduates came to Mark Sullivan, a journalist emeritus in the late 1930s, with letters of introduction.  They were seeking newspaper work.  He advised them that an "average career on a small-town paper ... may be more fruitful of satisfaction than an average career on a metropolitan newspaper."[11]  Chalmers Lowell Pancoast discovered that for himself after trying out for a job on the Cleveland Plain Dealer:

> During the week I wrote about drunks.  I covered fires.  I was sent to the Insane Asylum to write up their Christmas celebration.  I visited poverty-stricken families in the slums.  I called on aldermen, and chased "dogs and cats."  I went through the mill, seeing sordid things and learning sordid things, which gave me a different picture of life than I had received as a cub on a small town newspaper.[12]

Pancoast returned to the provinces with undisguised relief. Journalism there was a "big game ... something to enthuse over--to enjoy."  The young reporter was "looked up to--respected--his favors were courted....  He was given a freedom of privileges and expression which could never enter the life of a city cub."[13]

There was some truth in all this, but there was some illusion, too. Mark Twain mocked the notion that the country newspaper was especially pure. Twain had worked as a printer's devil on his older brother's weekly in Hannibal, Missouri. In the early 1860s, he was a reporter and editor on the Territorial Enterprise in Virginia City, Nevada. The frontier paper was an excellent classroom for the budding satirist. He was permitted to write what and how he wanted, and he produced squibs, burlesques, and hoaxes that gratified the town more than straight news.[14] From personal experience, Twain concluded that small-town journals were, in their own way, as irresponsible as city ones. The narrator of his humorous sketch "How I Edited an Agricultural Paper" declares with unconscious irony:

> I tell you I have been in the editorial business going on fourteen years, and it is the first time I ever heard of a man's having to know anything in order to edit a newspaper.... Who write the dramatic critiques for the second-rate papers? Why, a parcel of promoted shoemakers and apprentice apothecaries, who know just as much about good acting as I do about good farming and no more. Who review the books? People who never wrote one. Who do up the heavy leaders on finance? Parties who have had the largest opportunities for knowing nothing about it.... You try to tell me anything about the newspaper business! Sir, I have been through it from Alpha to Omega, and I tell you that the less a man knows the bigger the noise he makes and the higher the salary he commands.[15]

Writing under the pseudonym Paracelsus in Atlantic Monthly in 1902, a provincial editor alleged, "This ... is what a small newspaper does: it sells its space to the advertiser, its policy to the politicians." He further charged that readers in the hinterland craved sensationalism no less than those in the city. "Success came," he said, "when I exaggerated every little petty scandal, every row in a church choir, every hint of a disturbance. I compromised four libel suits and ran my circulation up to 3,200 in eleven months."[16]

William Allen White, owner-editor of the Emporia (Kan.) Gazette, romanticized life around a country newspaper shop in his collection of stories In Our Town (1906). In his autobiography, however, he described the country weeklies and small-town dailies of the 1880s and 1890s as "beggarly at best, and mendacious at worst. A newspaper was an organ sometimes political but, at bottom and secretly, an organ of some financial group which aimed at control of public utilities, or public patronage of one sort or other." White added that the country editor was often the "creature of his banker ... a pasteboard hero ... a disheveled, vain, discredited old pretender."[17]

The country newspaper of fiction--tolerant, personal, leisurely, and democratic--embodies qualities that were passing irretrievably out of journalism in the last quarter of the nineteenth century. White remarked that when he walked into the shabby office of the Eldorado (Kan.) Democrat in 1885 to learn newspapering, he had walked into a revolution, though he did not realize it then. Journalism was changing from an ancient craft into a business. The tools of the trade, such as cylinder presses and new types, were becoming expensive. Where once it required a few hundred dollars for a journeyman printer to start a paper, it now required a few thousand, an amount that was usually more than he could save.

His plight was shared by the shoemaker, the cabinet-maker, the wheelwright, the tanner, the saddler, and other craftsmen. "Machinery everywhere ... was dividing and multiplying," White said, "making new social, economic and political patterns, all based on the need for capital."[18] The country newspaper was fully a part of the complex modern world. Frank Luther Mott pointed out that between 1914 and 1940 the "movement for consolidation and mergers, the effects of the depression, and the trend toward independence of party were felt in rural and small city journalism quite as much as in that of the metropolitan centers."[19]

It was a fantasy that the countryside created simpler, happier lives. "Country life" novels appeared precisely at a time when the economic base of the United States was shifting from agriculture to industry. The village merchant saw business slipping away and his debts overcoming him. Towns and counties that had voted bonds for improvements--railroads, waterworks, electric lights, paved streets--went broke.[20] As the price of wheat tumbled below fifty cents a

bushel, and corn to twenty-eight cents, the farmer was driven
to the wall.  Over 11,000 farm mortgages were foreclosed in
Kansas alone from 1890 to 1894.  By 1900, one third of
American farmers were tenants.[21]

Against a background of financial panic, the Midwest
exploded in a Populist uprising.  Populism challenged the
prevailing ideologies of the period:  the success myth, social
Darwinism, and laissez-faire.[22]  "Debtors who could not pay,
overwhelmed with their personal calamities, each of which
seemed unique, were organizing with great vigor to redress
their wrongs,"[23] White recalled.  The fiction about country
journalism gave no inkling of the widespread turmoil.  Instead, it encouraged the daydream that somewhere beyond
the dirt and din of the city there was still a place un-
touched by the Industrial Revolution.  Within its pages,
people could escape the mounting problems of the present
and vicariously satisfy their nostalgia for a vanished golden
world.

The same images that appeared dark and twisted in
fiction set in the city room appeared curiously innocuous
and flat in the fiction set in the country newspaper office.
Freed from the urban maze, the journalist lost his ratlike
propensities.  The shadows in the portrait of the crusader,
the ambiguities in the portrait of the cub, were magically
erased.  What resulted were romances on the order of
White's In Our Town.

About 1904, White began writing the sketches that make
up the collection.  He sent a couple to George Horace Lorimer, editor of the Saturday Evening Post.  Lorimer asked
for more and paid a thousand dollars apiece for most of them.
"Each story was complete in form," White explained in his
autobiography, "yet all strung together as an account of
country newspapers in the eighties and nineties."  Published
in 1906, In Our Town had, in White's words, a "considerable
sale and more than passing vogue."  All the critics "reviewed
it with some enthusiasm."[24]

White's unnamed narrator, a folksy old reporter, describes the country newspaper as a "social clearing-house,"
where the editor and his staff "sooner or later pass upon
everything that interests their town."  They go about in
their shirt-sleeves, as it were, "calling people by their first

names; teasing the boys and girls good-naturedly; tickling
the pompous members of the village family, and letting out
the family secrets of the community without much regard
for the feelings of the supercilious." Small-town journalists
"get more than our share of fun out of life...," the narrator
says, "and pass as much of it on to our neighbors as we
can spare."[25] Newspaper work breeds in them an amused
tolerance, never cynicism or contempt. It is impossible to
imagine one remarking in the hard-boiled manner of star reporter Tim North, the protagonist of Malcolm H. Ross's
Penny Dreadful:

> We're so moral, so proud of our brilliant civilization.
> Tallest buildings in the world. Look at the Wool-
> worth tower over there--beautiful as a medieval
> prayer and stuffed with morons who ... satisfy
> their sex lives by reading the tabloids. It's a tab-
> loid civilization. And we're caught in it. Just try
> to escape! They're powerful as hell and about as
> witless.[26]

Metropolitan dailies pander to their readers; country
journals care for theirs. The compassion even extends to
competitors. Competition drives the urban press to bribery,
subterfuge, sensationalism, and fakery. Not the narrator's
newspaper. Its opposition, the Statesman, is run by General A. Jackson Durham, an "old buffalo horned out of the
herd." As befits the bucolic atmosphere of In Our Town,
the rivalry between the two papers is more hypothetical than
real. Occasionally, the general's foreman must borrow newsprint to publish the Statesman; "but they use so little,"
the narrator observes, "that we do not mind."[27] There is
no gloating over the fate of a fallen rival, only the offer
of a hand up, a gesture of sympathy unlikely to occur in
big-time journalism.

Newspaper work is regularly portrayed in fiction as
a cemetery of talent. Journalists on metropolitan papers
struggle and scheme to escape living burial. But death
came like a ministering angel for one of White's characters,
a reporter known as the Young Prince. After three years
of eating and sleeping with his work, he was struck down
by a fever and died--or, as White revealingly put it, "went
home."[28] The euphemism gilds tragedy with sunshine.
Evidently, life around a country newspaper office is so
placid that not even death can upset the equilibrium.

Wilbur Nesbit's The Gentleman Ragman (1906) similarly depicts small-town journalism as being protected from the shocks of reality by a golden aura. Nesbit wrote daily newspaper verse for many years, first on the Baltimore American and later on the Chicago Evening Post and the Chicago Tribune.[29] The narrator of his novel is a printer's devil, Johnny Thompson, for whom journalism is a school, though one in which he is taught very different things from his urban counterpart, the cub reporter.

When Jesse Lynch Williams's Billy Woods was a cub, he "had little to do with anything normal, because his job was to hunt and handle the News, which means the interesting, the unusual, surprising, shocking, remarkable, wonderful, wicked, horrible...."[30] His work took him into odd places and made him meet queer people. The education Johnny Thompson receives on a country newspaper is just the opposite--narrow and harmless. "[N]ow that I have learned to set type and write personal and local items for the weekly Chronicle," he says, "I have secured knowledge of a great many long words that will come in useful to me hereafter, in case I should decide to become a preacher, or maybe set up as a doctor."[31] Rural life imposes definite limits on what Johnny can experience: the limits of a dull propriety.

Removed to the countryside, the image of the crusading journalist also underwent an extraordinary transformation. The protagonist of Alice Hegan Rice's Mr. Opp (1909) launches the first paper ever in Cove City, a little Kentucky town that rests "serenely undisturbed by the progress of the world."[32] In this quiet setting, the whooping up of disaster and scandal that characterizes the metropolitan press would be anomalous. Opp's country weekly is a warm, kindly, reassuring presence:

> ... the front page of the "Eagle" was like the front
> door of a house; when once you got on the other
> side of it, you were in the family ... formality was
> dropped, and an easy atmosphere prevailed. You
> read that Uncle Enoch Siller had Sundayed over at
> the Bridge, or that Aunt Gussy Williams was on the
> puny list, and frequently there were friendly refer
> ences to "Ye Editor" or "Ye Quill Driver," for after
> soaring to dizzy heights in his editorials, Mr. Opp

condescended to come down on the second page and
move in and out of the columns, as a host among his
guests.[33]

The Eagle does scream for reforms, but what reforms!
Most newspaper crusaders in fiction battle potent evils--
vigilantes, gangsters, corrupt officials. Opp swats at nui-
sances. For example, he campaigns against the "right of
pigs to take their daily siesta in the middle of Main
Street...." His literal muckraking has appropriately quaint
effects. "The policies suggested by Mr. Opp, the editor,
were promptly acted upon by Mr. Opp, the citizen.... He
arranged a reform party and appointed himself leader....
In fact, he formed enough committees to manage a Presidential campaign."[34]

By the close of World War I, the sunny portrait of
country journalism had begun to cloud over. It was increasingly difficult to write pretty things after half the
world had gone up in flames. Henry Is Twenty (1918) by
Samuel Merwin, who had investigated Chicago meat packers
and the opium trade for Success magazine in the early 1900s,
looks critically at the small-town newspaper.[35] Although
set in the mid-1890s, the novel reflects some of the skepti-
cism and disillusionment of the postwar era.

Henry Calverly is a reporter on a weekly in the over-
grown village of Sunbury, Illinois. His is "curiously petty"
work, the "sort of job you associated with the off-time of
poor students." But Henry is not without ambition. He
aspires to be--no surprise--a writer. The novel treats with
gentle irony his efforts to free the "blazing artist" in him
from the "drifting, helpless youth."[36] There is nothing
gentle, however, about Merwin's treatment of journalism.

It is a sneaky, lying business. Henry finds that out
after he writes a tart account of the annual businessmen's
picnic. The owner of the Voice, afraid of offending readers
and advertisers, heavily censors the story. When Henry protests to the paper's editor, his friend Humphrey Weaver,
that he wrote the truth, he is told that was why it was re-
written. "Then they don't want the truth?" he naively asks.
"Good lord--no!" Humphrey exclaims.[37]

A frustrated Henry quits the Voice and joins its rival,

the Gleaner, run by Robert A. McGibbon, who once worked
on a yellow journal in New York. McGibbon has citified the
country newspaper. He "used bold-faced headings, touched
with irritating acumen on scandal, assailed the ruling political triumvirate, and made the paper generally fascinating
as well as disturbing." But big headlines do not sell papers
in small towns. McGibbon's energy and assertiveness "outraged every local prejudice ... alienated, one by one, each
friendly influence."38

He begs Henry to save his sinking paper. In three
days and nights of nearly nonstop writing, Henry dashes off
ten vivid, satiric pen-pictures of small-town life. Their
publication in the Gleaner creates a sensation, and Henry
is suddenly being compared to Kipling, Chaucer, Poe, and
the young Richard Harding Davis. After that, things happen fast--and with even greater disregard for logic and
reality.

Henry and Humphrey buy the Gleaner and turn it
around. Henry's sketches are reprinted in a national
magazine whose editor promises to publish them in book
form and make Henry famous within a year. And Henry
gets enough money from the deal to marry the girl of his
dreams.39 All of these developments are more or less as
expected in a popular romance. What is unexpected is how
caustically Merwin portrayed small-town journalism. Perhaps
the world war undermined the belief that beyond the horizon there was a place overflowing with virtue and happiness.
Merwin's novel is a transitional work, half in sunshine, half
in shadow. It shows the myth of innocence in the early
stages of decay.

The decay is more advanced in Sallie's Newspaper
(1924) by Edwin Herbert Lewis. Sallie Flowers is the beautiful young owner of the Seganku Daily Sun. After living
some years in California, she returns to her home town in
Wisconsin and proceeds to overhaul the paper her grand-
father founded. "I want everybody to know everybody else,
and learn to be charitable," she explains. Editor Jim
Fletcher is skeptical at first. When Sallie tells him to "take
all the news quietly" and avoid scareheads, he argues that
people "like to be scared."40

He ends up following Sally's instructions, not because

they make journalistic sense, but because he loves her. She orders that no display advertising be printed in the paper anymore. Advertisers could still send copy, only it would be presented as news and subject to revision. Her goal is "justice in advertising."[41] In the real world, the result would be bankruptcy.

But the Sun merely grows brighter. It operates under special dispensation. The small-town setting encloses the paper in a protective bubble. The bubble abruptly bursts when Lewis tosses into the plot the rape of a thirteen-year-old girl. This "awful disaster"[42] would have been unthinkable in the bland prewar fiction about country journalism, wherein sex was taboo. (One might have been excused for concluding that country folk reproduced by cell division.)

The rape does not wipe out the distinction between the country weekly or small-town daily and the city journal. A metropolitan paper would have exploited the incident in circulation-grabbing headlines. The Sun suppresses the story to shield the victim. It "did not sell a single extra on her account, or make a single cent out of her."[43]

And yet the crime marks the end of something. Sallie calls off her engagement to Jim and sails for England. Jim quits as editor to become a farmhand. Their noble journalistic experiment is abandoned. The fairy-tale enchantment that preserved the small town from change has been broken, perhaps never to be restored.

Fiction long portrayed country life as benign, and nowhere was the benignity better reflected than on the small newspaper. The very building that housed the paper breathed tranquility, sitting "like a contemplative old gentleman in its ancient and shabby garden" and watching with "mild interest the hasty world go by."[44] While the metropolitan daily was a circus and cynically fed the public's appetite for sensation, the country journal was a member of the village family and offered wise and caring counsel to its relations.

The picture probably contained an element of truth. In 1919, William Dudley Pelley, publisher-editor of the Caldenonian, an evening paper in St. Johnsbury, Vermont,

wrote in American Magazine that the country editor and his
readers "go down the hill of life together." "Your editor,
right in your home town," Pelley said, "probably knows more
good and bad about you than you ever dream he does. He
knows who are the liars and double-dealers and thieves and
scoundrels and four-flushers and horse-thieves in his community.... Yet his attitude toward them will doubtless be
a sort of amused tolerance. He has a lot of sympathy for
the ills to which human flesh is heir."[45]

That, however, was not the whole story. For decades,
fiction disguised what Iowa-bred William L. Shirer called the
"gray and narrow confines of rural civilization."[46] And it
ignored the social and economic revolution that was transforming country journalism from a craft into a business.
As William Allen White noted, the newspaper would become
"one of the major industries of every little town."[47]

The warm golden glow that surrounded the country
newspaper office in fiction finally began to fade after World
War I. No place seemed immune anymore from the contagion
of the twentieth century. I have found only one faint, fleet-
ing reference in contemporary newspaper novels to the old
myth of the countryside as sanctuary. The protagonist of
Herbert Mitgang's Kings in the Counting House (1983), an
unemployed reporter, says, "There are still papers around
that need pros to put them out, on the fringes of the city
if not in the city itself...."[48] Sunshine has given way to
shadow, innocence to experience. History has battered
down the gates of Eden.

## References

1. The newspaper movie, like the newspaper novel,
is usually set in the city. In fact, Dean Rossell observed
that the newspaper movie and the gangster movie were the
only film genres from the mid-1920s through the 1930s to
deal specifically with urban America. "It is with the gangster and the newshound, both vertically mobile through society, the one with his press pass, the other his gun,
where motion pictures intersected with an American society
changing from a rural culture to an urban one," Rossell
said. "Hollywood and the Newsroom," American Film, Vol.
I, no. 1, Oct. 1975, pp. 16-17.

2. Henry Justin Smith, Josslyn (Chicago: Covici-McGee, 1924), p. 43.

3. Commager, American Mind, p. 34.

4. Russel Nye, The Unembarrassed Muse (New York: Dial Press, 1970), p. 36.

5. Beer, Mauve Decade, p. 117.

6. Hart, Popular Book, p. 205.

7. Mott, American Journalism, p. 589.

8. Charles Moreau Harger, "The Country Editor of Today," The Profession of Journalism, p. 157.

9. Albert Blumenthal, Small-Town Stuff (Chicago: University of Chicago Press, 1932), p. 180.

10. Phillips, Great God Success, p. 28.

11. Mark Sullivan, The Education of an American (New York: Doubleday, Doran, 1938), pp. 115-16.

12. Chalmers Lowell Pancoast, Cub (New York: Devin-Adair, 1928), pp. 286-87.

13. Ibid., pp. 287-89.

14. Albert Bigelow Paine, Mark Twain, Vol. 1 (New York: Harper & Brothers, 1912), pp. 207-8.

15. Mark Twain, Editorial Wild Oats (New York: Harper & Brothers, 1905; reprint ed., New York: Arno Press, 1970), pp. 66-68.

16. Paracelsus, "Confessions of a Provincial Editor," The Profession of Journalism, pp. 141-42.

17. White, Autobiography, p. 126.

18. Ibid., pp. 126-27.

19. Mott, American Journalism, p. 729.

20. White, Autobiography, p. 215.

21. Commager, American Mind, p. 51.

22. Norman Pollack, The Populist Response to Industrial America (New York: Norton, 1962), p. 18.

23. White, Autobiography, p. 215.

24. Ibid., pp. 372-73.

25. William Allen White, In Our Town (New York: Macmillan, 1915), pp. 3, 6-7.

26. Ross, Penny Dreadful, p. 134.

27. White, In Our Town, pp. 143, 147.

28. Ibid., p. 27.

29. Mott, American Journalism, p. 584.

30. Williams, Stolen Story, p. 247.

31. Wilbur Nesbit, The Gentleman Ragman (New York: Harper & Brothers, 1906), pp. 1-2.

32. Alice Hegan Rice, Mr. Opp (New York: Century, 1909), p. 17.

33. Ibid., p. 103.

34. Ibid., pp. 204-5.

35. Kunitz and Haycraft, Twentieth Century Authors, p. 950; Lyon, Success Story, p. 238.

36. Samuel Merwin, Henry Is Twenty (Indianapolis: Bobbs-Merrill, 1918), pp. 80, 188.

37. Ibid., p. 165.

38. Ibid., pp. 236-37.

39. Henry Is Twenty is part of a trilogy. It was preceded by Temperamental Henry (1917), which Kunitz and Haycraft compared favorably to Booth Tarkington's Seventeen. It was followed by The Passionate Pilgrim (1919), which takes Henry into the impersonal, high-pressure world of big-city journalism.

40. Edwin Herbert Lewis, Sallie's Newspaper (Chicago: Hyman-McGee, 1924), pp. 35, 37.

41. Ibid., p. 37.

42. Ibid., p. 288.

43. Ibid.

44. Ray Stannard Baker [David Grayson], Hempfield (Toronto: Musson, 1915), pp. 10, 12. Baker first used the pseudonym David Grayson in 1906 for the series "Adventures in Contentment" in American Magazine. When the adventures were finished, the editors, as well as hundreds of readers, demanded more. Baker complied, and in a few years, David Grayson clubs sprang up around the country. Grayson's fame continued to spread after World War I as his stories began appearing in school anthologies. In all, Baker published nine Grayson books over thirty-five years. They sold a total of more than 2 million copies.

The fact that Grayson was Baker was a well-kept secret. It was not revealed until 1916 in an article in the Bookman. The secrecy reflected Baker's ambivalence toward his alter ego. Grayson provided a refuge from the social disorder he had witnessed as a muckraker for McClure's. A farmer-author, Grayson was quiet, optimistic, sentimental. Bannister, Ray Stannard Baker, pp. 112-14; Louis Filler, The Muckrakers (University Park: Pennsylvania State University Press, 1976), p. 348.

45. W. D. Pelley, "Human Nature As the Country Editor Knows It," American Magazine, Nov. 1919, pp. 60, 213.

46. William L. Shirer, 20th Century Journey (New York: Simon & Schuster, 1976), p. 156.

47. White, <u>Autobiography</u>, p. 313.
48. Herbert Mitgang, <u>Kings in the Counting House</u> (New York: Arbor House, 1983), p. 251.

Chapter V

## CONCLUSIONS

> I have let enough skeletons out of the
> newspaper closet. I will close the door and
> turn the key.
>
> > --A. E. Watrous, "The City
> > Editor"

The significance of newspaper fiction is multifaceted. First,
it is frequently a form of autobiography. Second, there is
anecdotal evidence that its protagonists served as role models
for young men and women aspiring to journalism careers.
Third, it reflected, and very likely helped shape, the public's image of the press. Fourth, it affords historians in-
sights into how journalists of the past felt toward their
work, as well as detailed descriptions of their work routine.

A critic in Philip Roth's novel The Anatomy Lesson
says, "... yes, I know there's a difference between characters and authors; I also know that grown-ups should not
pretend that it's quite the difference they tell their students
it is."[1] Throughout the previous pages, I have quoted the
words of characters as expressing the views of authors.
This is less foolhardy than it may appear at first. I have
taken, as Dorothy Burton Skaardal suggested one might,
the "recurrence of similar events, reactions, and ... moods
as evidence of validity...."[2] The incessant repetition of
certain themes over a span of forty years cannot entirely
be the result of coincidence. It bespeaks a commonality of
experience on the part of the authors, most of whom were
journalists-turned-novelists.

A good deal hinges on the question of whether newspaper fiction is autobiographical. If it is not, its significance as historical source material is severely limited. It
happens that the authors did draw heavily on their newspaper backgrounds. Within the context of popular literature, they recounted their bruising indoctrination in journalistic values and practices.

It has been said that "Nine times out of ten, a man
is the hero of his own stories."[3] Condy Rivers, the protagonist of Frank Norris's Blix: A Love Idyll, closely resembles his creator. Both Rivers and Norris were born in
Chicago and raised in San Francisco. Both lost their
fathers--Rivers by death, Norris by desertion. Both were
educated at state universities, then spent a year at an Ivy
League school--Rivers at Yale, Norris at Harvard. Both
returned to San Francisco, where they did hack work and
wrote self-consciously literary stories for local papers.
Last, both were called east to become editorial assistants
on magazines.[4]

One can cite endless examples of authors lightly fic-
tionalizing episodes from their journalism careers. David
Graham Phillips's experiences as a cub on the New York Sun
parallel those of Howard's on the News Record in The Great
God Success. Both became star reporters covering the same
"Lost Baby Found" story. Both listened to the cynical talk
of old newspapermen: "[T]hey say of other professions that
there is always room at the top. Journalism is just the re-
verse. The room is all at the bottom, no top--easy to enter,
hard to achieve, impossible to leave." And both evolved a
stoic philosophy: "Work and sleep--the two periods of un-
consciousness of self--are the two periods of happiness."[5]

Although the autobiographical strain in newspaper fiction is strong, fiction is not bound by truth as the word
is usually understood. Novels may be judged on many
criteria, but the degree of factual accuracy is not among
them. Authors have license to exaggerate and invent.
Paradoxically, by heightening and rearranging reality,
they unlock the secret meaning of things. The mind's eye
sees more than the naked eye.

As literary biographer Leon Edel explained, "Writers
create worlds for themselves in their books, they tell

parables, they offer allegories of the self. When they express these in the form of fiction or drama or poetry, we
have the work of a transfiguring imagination which uses
symbolic statement and myth to disguise autobiography."[6]
The allegories and parables of newspaper fiction are rela-
tively transparent. Journalists wrote novels about journalists who aspired to write novels and escape the grind of
daily journalism. In the process, they exorcised guilts,
vented fears, and rehearsed fantasies of retribution and
triumph.

Anxiety about the status of journalism runs like a
fault line through newspaper fiction, unsettling and crack-
ing the foundations, crumbling the image of journalists.
At every stage of its modern development, journalism has
been a target of criticism. The more popular it has become
in its appeals, the more strident the attacks from the educated classes. It has been accused of sensationalism, arrogance, greed, and worse. Denied public acknowledgment
of their prestige, journalists have lost faith that theirs is a
profession. Their insecurity is embodied in the portrayal
of journalism as either a school or a cemetery.

Harried by deadlines and haunted by self-doubt, fictional journalists seek to graduate to a more rewarding line
of work. Journalism is too superficial, too sordid, too
draining for them to think of staying in it indefinitely.
"[I]t's a darned small business for a grown man to go
scrutinizing the private lives of a lot of degenerates and
telling the world about them," a reporter grumbles in Ben
Ames Williams's Splendor.[7] Such cynicism is endemic to
newspaper fiction. "Always that note of despair; always
that pointing to the motto over the door of the profession:
'Abandon hope, ye who enter here.'"[8]

Yet the period 1890-1930 is generally assumed to have
been a golden age of journalism. These were the years
when press clubs sprang up, trade journals and journalism
textbooks appeared, and college instruction in journalism
got seriously under way. Samuel Blythe wrote in his mem-
oir, The Making of a Newspaper Man, that the era of the
"frowsy, alleged bohemian drunken reporter" was over.
"The present-day reporter," he asserted, "is an honorable,
clean, self-respecting man, working honorably and cleanly."[9]

That view is contradicted by newspaper fiction. It obsessively charted the emotional costs of a journalism career: disillusionment, drunkenness, decay, and death. Nowhere outside its pages can one find so comprehensive and consistent a record of the inner turmoil of journalists. Drawing on their personal experience, authors challenged the notion that journalism had smoothly progressed from a disreputable trade to a respectable profession. They lamented the long, irregular hours, the rush and strain, the prying into other people's affairs--"this gambling," as David Graham Phillips put it, "with our brains and nerves as the stake."[10]

Fiction provided journalists-turned-novelists with the freedom and form necessary to express the anxieties and insecurities they felt while grubbing on newspapers for a living. Of course, there were those who cunningly crafted their writing to what the literary market would bear. Even the most sincere and serious of the authors distorted to some extent. But "out of a pattern of lies," D. H. Lawrence said, "art weaves the truth."[11] Mere factual accuracy could never have conveyed as fully as the dark symbols and myths of newspaper fiction the horror of being buried alive in the cemetery of the city room.

In the 1935 movie Front Page Woman, a female cub arrives at a prison late one night to cover her first execution. When a veteran newspaperman from another paper voices surprise that she would request such a gruesome assignment, she snaps: "Why not? I'm a reporter." He smiles pityingly at her. "No, you're not," he says. "You're just a sweet little kid whose family allowed her to read too many newspaper novels."

In Adventure, Mystery, and Romance, John Cawelti referred to a friend who "has often remarked that all of us carry a collection of story plots in our heads and that we tend to see and shape life according to the plots."[12] In the early 1900s, young men and women aspiring to journalism careers sometimes got their image of newspaper work from fiction. All in all, it was not an image likely to instill idealism or build confidence. Yet they may have acted on the job the way they remembered fictional journalists acting.

When eighteen-year-old H. L. Mencken applied for a position on the Baltimore Morning Herald at the turn of the century, the "almost innumerable texts on journalism that now serve aspirants were ... unwritten...."[13] By default, he turned to newspaper fiction for guidance. He read Richard Harding Davis's "Gallegher," Elizabeth G. Jordan's Tales of the City Room (1898), and Jesse Lynch Williams's The Stolen Story and Other Newspaper Stories (1899).

Will Irwin was filled with misgivings on joining the reporting staff of the San Francisco Chronicle in 1900. During his college days, he had read "Gallegher" and The Stolen Story. He said the fiction "painted the newspaper reporter as a kind of superdetective who with preternatural acumen wrung their secrets from crooks, society women, and magnates in order to score sensational scoops."[14] Irwin doubted he was cut out for that sort of thing.

As a young reporter on the Milwaukee Sentinel, Lorena Hickock was entranced by Edna Ferber's Dawn O'Hara. Hickock, who was later a famous Associated Press correspondent, took to imitating Dawn's habit of drinking hot chocolate in an old German coffeehouse and steadily gained weight. The favorite girlhood reading of Mary Elizabeth Prim, a star reporter on the Boston Transcript in the 1930s, was Tales of the City Room.[15]

"The worst of it is," George Bernard Shaw complained, "when a spurious type gets into literature, it strikes the imagination of boys and girls. They form themselves by playing up to it; and thus the insubstantial fancies of one generation are apt to become the unpleasant and mischievous realities of the next."[16] Mark Sullivan was chagrined to discover that the college graduates who came to him each June for career advice thought of reporting "as they have seen it on the stage or in books."[17] The relationship between art and life is elusive, but not so elusive that the inspiration they take from each other is undetectable.

All the various types of newspapermen in fiction, from the would-be writer to the rum-soaked hack, were found in city rooms. "Any one who has worked in a newspaper office knows," John Macy said in 1922, "that the older men are likely to be weary and cynical and that the younger men fall into two classes, those who are too stupid to be discontented with any aspect of their position except the size of their salaries, and those who hope to rise to better paid positions, or to 'graduate,' as they put it, from daily journalism to other kinds of literary work."[18]

Fictional reporters will do almost anything for the sake of a story, including walking on water in the case of the protagonist in Ray Stannard Baker's "Pippins." Journalists actually followed a similar code. "'Get what you're sent for, if you have to go through fire and water,' is ... the injunction of the old hands to the new ones in journalism," Julian Ralph observed in 1903.[19] Economics created the relentless competition among papers. Fiction, however, helped spread and reinforce the image of the daring, ingenious, amoral newspaperman. Anecdotal evidence suggests that the youthful readers of newspaper novels who went on to journalism careers were the image made flesh.

At the same time, a number of journalists reacted with sarcasm and scorn to the image of the press in popular literature. Their jeering was a defense mechanism, for the image is, by and large, negative. David Shaw, media critic of the Los Angeles Times, has pointed out that journalists are terribly thin-skinned. "We don't like to be criticized," he wrote, "explicitly or implicitly, in print or on film, in truth or in fiction, anywhere or anytime by anyone. And when we are criticized ... we become even more sensitive, even more defensive, even more insistent that the portrayals are unfair, the criticism inaccurate."[20]

Malvina Lindsay, a reporter in Kansas City in the 1920s, noted that the "malcontent newspaper man, cursing a thankless calling and yet cleaving to it, is a prevailing figure in American fiction and drama." She derisively described how the "martyr journalist" is "invariably overworked, underpaid and unappreciated and in his old age is either ruthlessly kicked out or retained in the humiliating role of pensioner." It was with a certain bitter satisfaction that she concluded, "Nothing was ever more fortunate for the followers of a perilously overpopulated trade than this conception of the newspaper toiler...."[21]

Irvin S. Cobb was another who tried to drive a stake through the heart of the fictional journalist. In his autobiography, Exit Laughing, the comic novelist and former ace reporter exercised his heavy brand of humor on the character:

> Before the buoyant imaginations of moving-picture
> producers, as reflected on the silver screen, taught
> us that all great reporters were drunken geniuses,
> with a dashing way about them though, and that all
> women writers were beautiful abnormalities, and that
> a city room somewhat resembled feeding time at a
> zoo, a favorite fiction story was the one about the
> despised cub, whom even the copy boy snubbed and
> the Neroesque city editor sneered at and the rest of
> the staff ignored; but he went forth and all by him-
> self, through a superhuman stroke of brilliancy,
> outslicked the supercilious star of the opposition
> sheet right down to his union suit. This was known
> as a "scoop." Speaking personally, I never knew of
> but one such instance of success on the part of a
> comparative greenhorn when pitted against metropoli-
> tan talent. And success there was not to be attrib-
> uted to the young hero's intelligence. It was due
> to luck.[22]

The critics of newspaper fiction seem to have almost
intentionally misconstrued its purpose. A strictly factual
portrayal of journalism was not necessarily its primary goal--
or its goal at all. In George Gerbner's words, "To be true
to life in fiction would falsify the deeper truth of cultural
and social values served by symbolic functions."[23] The literary stereotypes of journalists survived as long as they
did because they struck an emotional chord in the public.
Yet the exact relationship between popular art and the
populace remains hidden. "[W]hat happens to the anonymous audience while it consumes the products of mass culture?" Irving Howe asked. "It is a question that can hardly
be answered systematically or definitively, for there is no
way of knowing precisely what the subterranean reactions
of an audience are...."[24]

But it would be odd if the image of journalism in fiction were unconnected to popular attitudes toward the press.
"I am constantly appalled anew," David Shaw commented,
"by how little otherwise intelligent, well-informed people
know about how a newspaper actually functions, about what
its objectives and limitations and traditions are, about its

structure and processes and its decision-making procedures."[25] Fiction, plays, television, and movies may be partly to blame for this. After seeing ten newspaper movies made between 1931 and 1974, New York Times critic Nora Sayre declared: "Small wonder that many moviegoers don't love or trust newspaper people; from the first film production of 'The Front Page' to the latest, over thirty years of movies have stated that reporters blithely invent the news while ignoring what really happened, and that the newsroom is a giant nursery seething with infantile beings."[26]

British literary historian Richard Hoggart claimed that to envision popular authors as consciously "compounding in just the right proportions all the various ingredients which go to make their success is ... to overestimate most of them." Rather, he said, they "possess some qualities in greater measure than their readers, but are of the same ethos. 'Every culture lives inside its own dream'; they share the common dream of their culture."[27] Americans dreamed in the pages of newspaper fiction that journalism both nurtured aspiring writers and destroyed their talent; stood up for the underdog and sold itself to the highest bidder; eschewed sensationalism and pandered to perverts and morons.

The contradictions reveal the love-hate relationship between the public and the press. From 1890 to 1930, the newspaper grew into a mass medium, and the techniques by which it achieved its spectacular growth were amusing and thrilling to some, baffling and shocking to others. The custodians of the status quo were the ones most disturbed by the new journalism. David Graham Phillips captured their uneasy reaction to the yellow journal in The Great God Success (1901):

> They read it as they never did before, because it interested them. They could not deny that what it said was true; that is, they could not deny it to their own minds, although they did vigorously deny it publicly. Those who were attacked directly or indirectly, or expected to be attacked, denounced the paper as an "outrage," a "disgrace to the city," a "specimen of the journalism of the gutter." Many who were assailed thought its course was "inexpedient," "tended to increase discontent among the lower classes," "weakened the influence of the better classes."[28]

Journalism was a revolutionary force, tearing up traditions, redefining public morality, and lending voice and encouragement to the disenfranchised. It reflected currents sweeping through every phase of American life. The skyrocketing circulations, the manic search for exclusive news, the sensational headlines, and the concentration of newspaper ownership were signs of an America changing from a rural society to an urban and industrial one. Since journalism so clearly mirrored and so loudly supported the new order, it became the preeminent symbol for the mechanization, standardization, democratization, and vulgarization of culture. The contradictory portrayal of journalists in fiction represents the extremes of what people hoped and feared amid the upheavals that accompanied the birth of the modern era.

The journalist was too controversial a figure in life to suddenly blossom into a satisfactory hero when placed between the covers of a book. "Certain professions have yielded few national idols," Dixon Wecter wrote in 1941.[29] He cited art, education, religion, medicine, and law; he might have added journalism if it were not so far down the list of possibilities as to be beneath mention.

John Cawelti pointed out that the "story of the newspaper reporter and the scoop" has "never had the sustained and widespread appeal of the western, the detective story, or the gangster saga." We witness the reporter filching pictures from the tops of dressers, asking embarrassing questions of tearful widows, cutting corners to beat competitors or meet deadlines, and bad-mouthing readers and editors in the barroom after work, and we recoil. "The pull of a literary formula," Cawelti said, "depends on audience identification with a hero who is typically better or more fortunate in some ways than ourselves."[30] The reporter is typically worse off in most ways than ourselves. He is driven, cynical, alcoholic, and unfulfilled.

The public basically got the kind of portrayal of the press it demanded. Confused and threatened by the pace and direction of social change, people needed both a savior and a scapegoat, and the journalist, a leading actor in the drama of the modern world, could be made to fill either role. Sometimes he was a messiah who appeared out of nowhere to solve problems a community was incapable of solving for itself. But more often, he was a frustrated hack with indecent and unnatural ideas in his head, whisky on his breath, no money in his pocket, and the gutter before him.

Newspaper fiction is part autobiography and part wish-fulfillment fantasy. On both counts, it is potentially of interest to historians. It shows how the first generation of modern journalists felt about their work and how the public felt about these modern journalists. What it offers is a symbolic and subjective account of journalism in the last decade of the nineteenth century and the early decades of the twentieth. The characters may be wooden, and the plots melodramatic. Yet, as Grant C. Knight suggested, "it is necessary for an understanding of culture to know not only what people should have read but also what they did read."[31] Popular literature constitutes a kind of diary of the attitudes and tensions and dreams of the society that produced and consumed it.[32]

Authors of fiction are trespassers. They sneak about the secret--and, in the case of newspaper fiction, foggy--landscape of the heart. Not all explore it to the same depth or with the same sense of discovery. But even the dullest generally bring back something intriguing. Their choice of a particular hero or villain may unconsciously reveal their preoccupations and yearnings, or those of their readers, or both. In this regard, newspaper fiction can refine our picture of journalism history. It divulges the inside story, exposes the hidden costs of visible progress.

Some, perhaps most, historians are instinctively hostile to the notion of fiction as a historical source. One labeled it "simply a crock." "Common sense tells you," he said, "that fiction writers are not bound by truth--that is why it is called fiction--but rather write what interests people and what they want to read.... [I]t's ridiculous to suppose that we can trust fiction to tell us anything beyond the fictional view ... at one particular point in time."[33] It is no more ridiculous, however, than supposing that we can trust newspapers, letters, memoirs, and histories to tell us the actual view. William Allen White admitted in the preface to his autobiography that the book, "in spite of all the pains I have taken and the research I have put into it, is

necessarily fiction." He warned readers "not to confuse
his story with reality. For God only knows the truth."[34]
Life is too hurried and situations too intricate for us to see
more than a fragment of the truth, and the problem is com-
pounded when dealing with events that occurred in a world
now gone to dust. The biggest part of the "truth" must always be pieced together in our imaginations.

"Art," D. H. Lawrence said, "has two great functions.
First, it provides an emotional experience. And then, if
we have the courage of our own feelings, it becomes a mine
of practical truths. We have had the feelings ad nauseam.
But we've never dared dig the actual truth out of them, the
truth that concerns us...."[35] The emotions attached to
the story patterns and stereotypes of newspaper fiction are
dark and unpleasant. For the sake of the reputation of the
press, they would best be left buried, and so, have been.

Fiction portrays journalism as a "strange world where
brilliant young men turn out to be sad old men."[36] Newspaper work was not a career but either a steppingstone to
something else or a cemetery. "Business'll kill you if you
keep on," the city editor in Henry Justin Smith's Deadlines
(1923) advises a cub. "Look at me, hauled out of bed at
five every morning; rush to my desk, stay there till the
last dog's hung. Fight, fight, fight, all the time. Fight
with the staff, with the readers of the paper, with the town
itself.... Get a quieter job, where you can write those
poems of yours. Nothing in this boiler-shop grind...."[37]

Reporters and editors wasted their energy on an
"evanescent product, forgotten as soon as made."[38] A newspaper was a mass of distractions and delusions, in large
measure because readers wanted to be distracted and de-
luded. "Spice: that's what we're looking for," an old newspaperman says in Samuel Hopkins Adams's Success. "Something to tickle their jaded palates. And they despise us
when we break our necks or hearts to get it for 'em." In
the face of such hypocrisy, journalists grow bitter and
cynical. "The men who go to the top in journalism, the big
men of power and success and grasp, come through with a
contempt for the public which they serve, compared to which
the contempt of the public for the newspaper is as skim milk
to corrosive sublimate."[39]

What common sense tells us is not all there is to tell. The dark imaginings contained in newspaper fiction were the shadows of real fears and doubts. Throughout the period when journalism was assuming some of the trappings of a profession, journalists-turned-novelists were recalling the terrors of newspaper life and echoing public worries about the sensational, profit-hungry press. The unflattering image did not appear accidentally but had specific causes. And while it is possible to disagree on these, it seems indisputable that forty years of bad dreams amount to rather more than sheer escapism.

On a less abstract level, historians can find valuable information in the background details of newspaper fiction. The authors, speaking from firsthand experience, described the procedures that journalists followed in gathering and processing the news. Their descriptions occasionally sound surprisingly modern. Here is legislative reporter Billy Gutherie of Joseph A. Altsheler's Gutherie of the Times haggling with a source:

> "Billy," said Warfield, "if I give you an important piece of news, will you pledge your word not to use it to-night?"
> "Are you sure that I could not get it except from you?"
> "Quite sure."
> "I'm released from my promise, if anybody else should come to me of his own volition and tell it to me?"
> "Certainly."
> "All right; I promise. What is it?"[40]

The impact of industrialization on journalism has often been discussed by historians, but not in the negative terms used by fiction writers. Fiction indicates just how bewildering the transformation of the newspaper office into a factory was. Stephen French Whitman, who worked as a reporter on the New York Evening Sun, vividly re-created the nightmarish atmosphere on a large, metropolitan daily in his naturalistic novel Predestined. The passage is worth quoting in full:

> From the second story, where he saw nothing but rough partitions and closed doors, Felix mounted by

a flight of spiral iron steps that ran up through a
gloomy shaft. He smelled dust, steam, hot metal.
A persistent, heavy rumbling seemed to make the
whole building tremble. Suddenly, close behind
him, downward dropped a freight elevator laden with
men in grimy undershirts. He was next startled
by the shrill scream of a circular saw, and, looking
below, through the interstices of the staircase he
perceived, as if at the bottom of a well, a confusion
of machinery, fires, caldrons of molten metal, half-
naked figures glistening with sweat.... Finally, he
emerged into a large room floored with iron plates.
Youths in leather aprons were rolling ponderous,
table-like objects back and forth or running about
with steaming mats of felt. Beyond these a swarm
of men were engaged in various peculiar perform-
ances. To the left, some, with armfuls of metal
spools, were walking between lines of small, racket-
ing machines. To the right, others, wearing eyeshades, were standing before type-cases. Ahead,
some distance off, among a huddle of desks, in a
fog of tobacco smoke, reporters in their shirt-
sleeves were writing, calling out to one another,
waving above their heads large sheets of paper,
which boys snatched from their hands and scurried
off with.[41]

Silence on a subject can be nearly as revealing to historians as emotionally charged language. There is no mention of the First Amendment in the newspaper fiction published from 1890 to 1930. Both in and out of fiction, journalists thought of their work as a game or racket, not a
responsibility. "[V]ery few of us would have remained,
year after year, in various newspaper jobs if we had felt
we could not treat it as a game," Vernon McKenzie observed
in 1931. "This is one of the compensations for inadequate
salaries and eccentric hours."[42] Billy Gutherie had been a
lawyer, but he found that the "law did not interest him a
particle...." Reporting, by contrast, "was like a game of
base-ball, played for its own sake--for the game itself."[43]

Veteran players shunned the title journalist. It was
too pretentious and implied a higher professional status than
they sought or deserved. Only misguided cubs persisted in
using it. Others preferred the less imposing newspaperman.

"[Y]ou see," the city editor explains to the young hero of
Edward Hungerford's The Copy Shop, "we are not aiming
to make a journalist of you.... If we can make an every-
day all-around newspaperman out of you..., we shall think
that there's a crown of glory for us somewhere."[44] When
Ray Stannard Baker's Pippins confides to a seasoned reporter his ambition to become a "great journalist," he is
answered with a "grim smile."[45] He has yet to realize that
good feet count for more in journalism than intellect.

"We are told about the world before we see it," Walter
Lippmann wrote. "We imagine most things before we experience them. And those preconceptions ... govern the whole
process of perception." He added that the bluenoses "who
wish to censor art do not at least underestimate this influence.... [T]hey feel vaguely that the types acquired
through fiction tend to be imposed on reality."[46] Historians
of American journalism usually lack a similar feeling. They
share with journalists--perhaps because many were journalists themselves at one time--a notion of truth limited to what
is attributable, palpable, or quantifiable. Of "strange brutes
of some forgotten dream" and "old prejudices submerged and
shadowy in the mind that reads," they have no proof, as
they narrowly define it.[47]

Newspaper fiction planted preconceptions in the mind
or reflected and reinforced preconceptions already there.
The preconceptions became as iron bars that imprisoned the
journalist. He may have been a willing prisoner of his fictional image, but even if he were not, the public would have
still seen him through the bars of a stereotype. For, to
paraphrase Keats, fiction is truth, truth fiction--that is all
we know on earth.

The moods and themes of newspaper fiction have demonstrated a remarkable staying power. Except for the idyll
of country journalism, they have continued into the 1980s.
The rise of radio and television, with their wider reach and
stronger emotional pull than the mass-circulation daily, has
actually sharpened the paranoia and guilt that have characterized the image of journalists from the outset.

Rather than heralds of a new, more enlightened age
of journalism, the electronic media are portrayed as having

brought yellow techniques to their logical--and disheartening--conclusion. The point is repeatedly made in contemporary novels that those on TV "aren't journalists, they're actors and actresses." John Denson, private eye, former newspaperman, and narrator of Richard Hoyt's 30 for a Harry (1981), elaborates: "The network people give us an almost unrelieved diet of shootings in Belfast, kidnappings in Rome, and skirmishes in Beirut with an oversimplified report by an economics reporter thrown in to justify it as news. It's show business ... no place for anybody with brains."[48]

Television demands "shattering pictures of violence and its victims, demands riots, fires, disasters, death, each picture more horrible than the last to stir even an instant of emotion." The protagonist of Barbara Gordon's Defects of the Heart (1983), a documentary filmmaker for a public-TV station in New York, initially blames sensationalism on an audience that "can respond only to blatant suffering, exaggerated outrage." But she is seized by an "even grimmer truth" while filming a documentary about a drug suspected of causing birth defects. She catches herself wishing that one of the young casualties were more damaged than he is, that he and his parents were not so cheerful and accepting. "What kind of woman am I, what kind of woman have I become, that I am disappointed not to find this family drowning in despair?" she wonders. "What have I done to feed the monstrous maw of television? How could I have thought I would have a better film if Timmy really were a monster? I am the monster."[49]

Whether working for TV or newspapers, most characters are guided by "professional opportunism."[50] They do not turn down a hot story, though it undermines their integrity and threatens the well-being of the public. Malcolm Anderson, a Miami reporter who loses his objectivity and nearly his life tracking a serial murderer in John Katzenbach's In the Heat of the Summer (1982), had frankly predicted:

> No matter how many people this guy kills, no matter how sickening the crimes are, no matter how closely connected we are to the acts themselves, the paper will always pursue the story. We can't do anything

else. We're not equipped to react like a responsible
organization, like a bureaucracy or the police.
Things happen, we write stories.... We're just
lucky that crazy people like this killer come along
every so often to help us do our job.[51]

"Sometimes I think I'm a parasite," a newspaper pho-
tographer in Katzenbach's novel says. "We all are."[52] And
yet, they, too, are preyed upon. Corporations have invaded journalism and reduced the journalist to a "wage-
earning servant, as impotent and unimportant, considered
as an individual, as a mill-hand."[53] He may have the duty
to write the truth, but he does not often have the opportunity. "What do you call people like us who have to work
for the black hats or not at all?" a reporter asks in Herbert
Mitgang's Kings in the Counting House.[54] The answers one
could give would not be very inspiring.

Alarm over the centralization of newspaper ownership
has been reflected in fiction since the first decade of the
twentieth century. There began appearing then lurid portraits of ruthless press lords, such as Howard in David
Graham Phillips's The Great God Success and David Holman
in William R. Hereford's The Demogog. As concentrated
ownership has increased--today "fifty corporations own most
of the output of daily newspapers and most of the sales and
audience in magazines, broadcasting, books, and movies"--
so has fear that the public is being brainwashed.[55] The
men who control the media are portrayed as amoral at best,
criminally insane at worst. They have no love for journalism or faith in the people. They are devoted solely to their
selfish interests. As is said of the publisher in 30 for a
Harry:

Harold has never worked in the newspaper; he's
never written or edited a story. He's never made
a decision about the news. He likes it because of
status and wealth. He likes it because he's on a
first-name basis with governors and United States
senators. He likes the parties and junkets. He
likes the power.[56]

Power, as Irving Wallace put it with characteristic
delicacy in The Almighty (1982), is the "ultimate orgasm."

A mad quest for power leads his protagonist, Edward Armstead, to pay a terrorist organization to create exclusive
stories for his newspapers and TV stations. After he has
scooped the competition on a string of spectacular crimes
staged by the gang, he raves, "I am the news. I make the
news. I make life that goes on in the world."57

Armstead is undone by one of his own investigative
reporters. Contemporary novels follow a long literary tradition in presenting a split image of journalism. The paranoid
fantasy of the press lord who literally kills for circulation
is balanced by the heroic myth, launched back in the Progressive Era, of the crusading journalist who identifies with
the weak and persecuted. In America of the 1980s, where
far-reaching decisions are made by invisible bureaucrats,
the economy is either staggering out of a crisis or stumbling
into one, and the future is threatened by nuclear war, the
reading public needs to lean on the strength of the crusader
more than ever.

"There are no accidents--that assumption is at the
root of political paranoia," a student of the phenomenon has
written. It is also at the root of recent fiction about journalism. The novels are mainly thrillers, and between gro-
tesquely detailed descriptions of sex and violence, they
portray "news and even history itself as a stage play to
amuse the masses while the real events transpire in secrecy."58 Everything is a lie. No one is what he seems.
The philanthropist is a cutthroat, the patriot a traitor.

This can be strangely comforting. The fiction explains away the social chaos of our times as the work of a
handful of conspirators, and so absolves the rest of us.
A clear, consistent pattern suddenly emerges from the bewildering headlines about assassinations, race riots, oil
shortages, and White House scandals. "Conspiracies do
exist, my friend," a KGB agent assures the hero--and, of
course, the readers--of Bill Granger's Schism (1981).
"Even if you must make a joke of them."59

It is not the establishment press that uncovers the
conspiracies. Exposure is accomplished by those on the
fringes of journalism: a struggling free-lancer, an unknown
cub, an old reporter thrown onto the street when his paper
dies. The media have been penetrated by the conspirators,

and maverick journalists must fight even their colleagues to get the truth out to the public. In Kings in the Counting House, the truth never is told. Protagonist Sam Linkum, who happens upon a conspiracy involving communication satellites, a TV network, oil and mineral resources, Saudi Arabians, and the Pentagon, can only wish that "there were a newspaper around that could unravel the connections and print the whole story...."[60]

The authors ritualistically invoke the memory of the Watergate affair. "A high school graduate and a Yalie with a reputation as a bum writer brought down the President of the United States. It is the stuff of myth," the narrator of 30 for a Harry says.[61] After the hero of Arnaud de Borchgrave and Robert Moss's The Spike (1980) exposes a Soviet plot to conquer the West with "disinformation," he is congratulated for the "best piece of enterprise journalism since Woodward and Bernstein brought down Nixon."[62] Ironically, what the references to Watergate seem most to suggest is that the press rarely lives up to its stated ideals and then only through the quixotic investigative reporter. Suspicion of journalism as an institution runs deep in the novels. There are too many one-newspaper towns, too many frightening stories broadcast over the airwaves and emblazoned in print, too many controversial court cases concerning anonymous sources, libel, and the right to privacy, for it to be otherwise. Bob Woodward, now an editor on the Washington Post, has himself remarked: "People are not going to look at the press normally as their friend. My feeling always is that we're outsiders. The period of the mid-70's may have been a little different, but it wasn't a natural situation."[63]

To be treated as prostitutes and parasites when they want to be treated as professionals erodes the enthusiasm of the better class of journalists. They ask for public acknowledgment of their prestige, but they receive public scorn. Shaken, they begin to wonder whether journalism is a career or a catch-basin for failures and misfits. A national survey conducted in 1971 found that "between a fifth and a quarter of experienced young editorial personnel in the news media ... seriously question their commitment to remain in the field.... [I]t would appear to be the most qualified who most seriously entertain thoughts of leaving."[64]

As in the past, anxiety about the social standing of journalism is reflected today in its portrayal as either a school or a cemetery. Journalists in fiction continue to bemoan the lack of reward in newspaper work. They enter it seeking romance or glory or experience and emerge a short time later alcoholic, cynical, and neurotic:

> The people out there are crying, laughing, bleeding, dying, and lying. It doesn't take a reporter long, not long at all, to know the awful, unbearable truth. And so across the land they sit in the bar next door hunkered down under the weight of their burden and swap callous, barbarous, outrageous stories of life in the city. These are men who know that God is, in fact, dead.[65]

Old reporters still warn newcomers to get out of journalism before it is too late. "[T]he newspaper business is miserable," one tells a female cub in The Almighty. "No place for a decent young lady. It makes you devious, hypocritical, immoral. It makes you forget people are human beings with feelings. It makes you warp the truth for stories."[66] The working life of the journalist is short, nasty, and brutish. In Philip Caputo's DelCorso's Gallery (1983), wire service correspondent Harry Bolton declares, "I don't want to finish as a fifty-year-old bureau bum, gone in the legs and winging stories until some young wolf comes along and takes my job, hell, I'm only thirty-six and already I'm winging it."[67] He resigns and retreats to a mountain cabin to write novels. The choice is ever flight or death.

Born in the age of clattering Linotypes, editors in green eyeshades, and ragged newsboys hawking extras on street corners, newspaper fiction has survived into our own age of media events, computerized newsrooms, and backyard satellite dishes with its original images and motifs more or less intact. Through one revolution after another in the technology for gathering, processing, and delivering the news, the hopes and doubts of journalists, as embodied in popular literature, have remained fairly constant. They still fear creative blight, still resent their status as social outcasts, still long for vindication.

Myths endure because they organize experience into interesting and agreeable patterns. Newspaper fiction represents more than the disillusioned views of journalists. It represents the necessary illusions of the public at large. Amid the pain and confusion of modern existence, literary stereotypes fulfill the poignant human need for identifiable heroes and villains. Popular imagination has invested journalism, which has told the calamitous history of the past century in shocking headlines and measured out our lives in column inches, with inordinate power to do good or evil. Journalists have been portrayed by turns as idealists and hardened cynics, crusaders and midnight conspirators. Our attitude toward them continually swings from dark to bright and back again. The cub who fumbles a story, the star who scores a scoop, the sob sister who betrays a source, the press lord who slants the news: These are figures borrowed from reality and set down within a half-soothing, half-terrifying dream from which there is no awaking.

## References

1. Philip Roth, The Anatomy Lesson (New York: Farrar, Straus, & Giroux, 1983), p. 85.
2. Skaardal, "Immigrant Literature," p. 15.
3. Leonard Burt, the late chief detective of Scotland Yard, quoted in Time, Sept. 19, 1983, p. 102.
4. Hart, Novelist in the Making, p. 23.
5. Phillips, Great God Success, pp. 9, 93; Ravitz, David Graham Phillips, pp. 31-33, 40, 42.
6. Leon Edel, The Stuff of Sleep and Dreams: Experiments in Literary Psychology (New York: Avon Books, 1982), p. 60.
7. Williams, Splendor, p. 361.
8. Phillips, Great God Success, p. 17.
9. Blythe, Making of a Newspaper Man, p. 238.
10. Phillips, Great God Success, p. 12.
11. D. H. Lawrence, Studies in Classic American Literature (New York: Viking Press, 1964), p. 2.
12. John Cawelti, Adventure, Mystery, and Romance (Chicago: University of Chicago Press, 1976), p. 24.
13. Mencken, Choice of Days, p. 142.
14. Irwin, Making of a Reporter, p. 31.
15. Ishbel Ross, Ladies of the Press (New York: Harper & Brothers, 1936), pp. 205, 486.
16. Quoted in Beer, Mauve Decade, p. 153.
17. Sullivan, Education of an American, p. 116.

18. Macy, "Journalism," p. 40.

19. Ralph, Making of a Journalist, p. 34.

20. David Shaw, "On Arrogance and Accountability in the Press," address presented at the University of Hawaii, March 8, 1983, p. 7.

21. Lindsay, "Jackdaw in Peacock's Feathers," p. 192.

22. Irvin S. Cobb, Exit Laughing (Indianapolis: Bobbs-Merrill, 1941; reprint ed., Detroit: Gale Research, 1974), pp. 96-97.

23. George Gerbner, "Teacher Image and the Hidden Curriculum," American Scholar, Winter 1972-1973, p. 69.

24. Irving Howe, "Notes on Mass Culture," Mass Culture, ed. by Bernard Rosenberg and David Manning White (Glencoe, Ill.: Free Press, 1960), p. 498.

25. Shaw, "On Arrogance and Accountability," p. 7.

26. Nora Sayre, "Falling Prey to Parodies of the Press," Jan. 1, 1975, New York Times Encyclopedia of Film, 1975-76 (New York: Times Books, 1984), unpaged.

27. Richard Hoggart, The Uses of Literacy (London: Chatto & Windus, 1957), pp. 172-73.

28. Phillips, Great God Success, p. 182.

29. Dixon Wecter, The Hero in America (New York: Scribner's, 1941), p. 477.

30. Cawelti, Adventure, Mystery, and Romance, pp. 18, 20.

31. Knight, Critical Period in American Literature, p. viii.

32. For more on this point, see William O. Aydelotte, "The Detective Story as a Historical Source," Yale Review, Sept. 1949-June 1950, pp. 76-95.

33. Personal letter to author from anonymous referee of Association for Education in Journalism and Mass Communication (History Division) papers competition, May 1985.

34. White, preface to Autobiography, no p.

35. Lawrence, Studies in Classic American Literature, p. 2.

36. Ross, Penny Dreadful, p. 62.

37. Henry Justin Smith, Deadlines (Chicago: Covici-McGee, 1923), p. 193.

38. Ibid., p. 111.

39. Adams, Success, p. 282.

40. Altsheler, Gutherie of the Times, p. 94.

41. Whitman, Predestined, pp. 53-54.

42. Vernon McKenzie, ed., Behind the Headlines (New York: Jonathan Cape & Harrison Smith, 1931), p. xi.

43. Altsheler, Gutherie of the Times, pp. 4-5.

44. Hungerford, Copy Shop, p. 32.

45. Baker, "Pippins," p. 435.

46. Walter Lippmann, Public Opinion (New York: Free Press, 1965), pp. 59-60.

47. Beer, Stephen Crane, p. 239.

48. Richard Hoyt, 30 for a Harry (New York: M. Evans, 1981), pp. 166-67.

49. Barbara Gordon, Defects of the Heart (New York: Harper & Row, 1983), p. 180.

50. Arnaud de Borchgrave and Robert Moss, Monimbó (New York: Simon & Schuster, 1983), p. 31.

51. John Katzenbach, In the Heat of the Summer (New York: Ballantine, 1982), pp. 110-11.

52. Ibid., p. 127.

53. Macy, "Journalism," pp. 36-37.

54. Mitgang, Kings in the Counting House, p. 220.

55. Ben H. Bagdikian, The Media Monopoly (Boston: Beacon Press, 1983), p. xvi.

56. Hoyt, 30 for a Harry, pp. 148-49.

57. Irving Wallace, The Almighty (Garden City, N.Y.: Doubleday, 1982), pp. 95, 313.

58. George Johnson, Architects of Fear: Conspiracy Theories and Paranoia in American Politics (Los Angeles: Jeremy P. Tarcher, 1983), pp. 24-25.

59. Bill Granger, Schism (New York: Crown, 1981), p. 153.

60. Mitgang, Kings in the Counting House, p. 219.

61. Hoyt, 30 for a Harry, p. 41.

62. Arnaud de Borchgrave and Robert Moss, The Spike (New York: Crown, 1980), p. 369.

63. Quoted in Jane Gross, "Movies and the Press Are an Enduring Romance," New York Times, June 2, 1985, sec. 2, p. 19.

64. John W. C. Johnstone, Edward J. Slawski, and William W. Bowman, The News People: A Sociological Portrait of American Journalists and Their Work (Urbana: University of Illinois Press, 1976), p. 154.

65. Hoyt, 30 for a Harry, p. 29.

66. Wallace, Almighty, p. 44.

67. Philip Caputo, DelCorso's Gallery (New York: Holt, Rinehart, & Winston, 1983), p. 310.

# BIBLIOGRAPHY

Newspaper Fiction, 1890-1930

Adams, Samuel Hopkins. The Clarion. New York: Grosset & Dunlap, 1914.

_____. Common Cause. Boston: Houghton Mifflin, 1919.

_____. Success. Boston: Houghton Mifflin, 1921.

Altsheler, Joseph A. Gutherie of the Times. New York: Doubleday, Page, 1904.

Baker, Ray Stannard [David Grayson]. Hempfield. Toronto: Musson, 1915.

_____. "Pippins." Youth's Companion, Sept. 7, 1899, pp. 435-36.

Beach, Rex. The Iron Trail. New York: Harper & Brothers, 1913.

Brooks, Jonathan. See Mellett, John C.

Brush, Katharine. Young Man of Manhattan. New York: Farrar & Rinehart, 1930.

Claudy, Carl H. The Girl Reporter. Boston: Little, Brown, 1930.

Cline, Leonard. Listen, Moon! New York: Viking Press, 1926.

Cobb, Irvin S. _Alias Ben Alibi_. New York: George H. Doran, 1925.

Comfort, Will Levington. _Red Fleece_. New York: George H. Doran, 1915.

Crane, Stephen. _Active Service_. New York: International Association of Newspapers & Authors, 1901.

_____. _Wounds in the Rain_. London: Methuen, 1900.

Davis, Elmer. _Friends of Mr. Sweeney_. New York: Robert M. McBride, 1925.

Davis, Richard Harding. "A Derelict," _Ransom's Folly_. New York: Scribner's, 1904.

_____. _The Deserter_. New York: Scribner's, 1917.

_____. _Gallegher and Other Stories_. New York: Scribner's, 1904.

_____. "The Red Cross Girl." _Saturday Evening Post_, March 2, 1912, pp. 3-6, 44-46.

_____. "The Reporter Who Made Himself King," _The King's Jackal_. New York Scribner's, 1904.

Dell, Floyd. _The Briary-Bush_. New York: Knopf, 1921.

_____. _Moon Calf_. New York: Knopf, 1920.

Dodge, Louis. _Whispers_. New York: Scribner's, 1920.

Dreiser, Theodore. "Nigger Jeff" and "A Story of Stories," _Free and Other Stories_. New York: Boni & Liveright, 1918.

Eggleston, George Cary. _Blind Alleys_. Boston: Lothrop, Lee & Shepard, 1906.

Ferber, Edna. _Cimarron_. Greenwich, Conn.: Fawcett, 1971.

_____. _Dawn O'Hara_. New York: Grosset & Dunlap, 1911.

Fergusson, Harvey. Capitol Hill. New York: Knopf, 1923.

Fowler, Gene. Trumpet in the Dust. New York: Liveright, 1930.

Gilson, Roy Rolfe. Miss Primrose. New York: Harper & Brothers, 1906.

Grayson, David. See Baker, Ray Stannard.

Harrison, Henry Sydnor. Queed. Boston: Houghton Mifflin, 1911.

Hart, James S., and Byrnes, Garrett D. Scoop. Boston: Little, Brown, 1930.

Hecht, Ben. Erik Dorn. New York: Putnam's, 1921; reprint ed., Chicago: University of Chicago Press, 1963.

Hereford, William Richard. The Demagog. New York: Henry Holt, 1909.

Hough, Clara Sharpe. Not for Publication. New York: Century, 1927.

Hungerford, Edward. The Copy Shop. New York: Putnam's, 1925.

Jordan, Elizabeth G. Tales of the City Room. New York: Scribner's, 1898.

Kelland, Clarence Budington. Contraband. New York: A. L. Burt, 1923.

Levin, Meyer. Reporter. New York: John Day, 1929.

Lewis, Edwin Herbert. Sallie's Newspaper. Chicago: Hyman-McGee, 1924.

Locke, William J. Jaffery. New York: John Lane, 1915.

London, Jack. "Amateur Night," Moon Face and Other Stories. New York: Macmillan, 1906.

Lorimer, George Horace. The False Gods. New York: Appleton, 1906.

Lyman, Olin L. Micky. Boston: Richard G. Badger, 1905.

MacLean, Charles Agnew. The Mainspring. Boston: Little, Brown, 1912.

Matthews, Brander. "An Interview with Miss Marlenspuyk," Outlines in Local Color. New York: Scribner's, 1921.

Mellett, John C. [Jonathan Brooks]. High Ground. Indianapolis: Bobbs-Merrill, 1928.

_____. Ink. Indianapolis: Bobbs-Merrill, 1930.

Merwin, Samuel. Henry Is Twenty. Indianapolis: Bobbs-Merrill, 1918.

_____. The Passionate Pilgrim. Indianapolis: Bobbs-Merrill, 1919.

_____. Temperamental Henry. Indianapolis: Bobbs-Merrill, 1917.

Michelson, Miriam. Anthony Overman. New York: Doubleday, Page, 1906.

_____. A Yellow Journalist. New York: Appleton, 1905.

Nesbit, Wilbur. The Gentleman Ragman. New York: Harper & Brothers, 1906.

Norris, Frank. Blix: A Love Idyll. In A Novelist in the Making. Ed. by James D. Hart. Cambridge: The Belknap Press/Harvard University Press, 1970.

Noyes, Alfred. "May Margaret," Walking Shadows. New York: Frederick A. Stokes, 1918.

Otis, Alexander. Hearts Are Trumps. New York: John McBride, 1909.

Paine, Albert Bigelow. The Breadline: A Story of a Paper. New York: Century, 1900.

Pancoast, Chalmers Lowell. "Scoops." Blue Book, Nov. 1906, pp. 196-201.

Phillips, David Graham. The Great God Success. New York: Grosset & Dunlap, 1901; reprint ed., Ridgewood, N.J.: Gregg Press, 1967.

————. A Woman Ventures. New York: Grosset & Dunlap, 1902.

Rice, Alice Hegan. Mr. Opp. New York: Century, 1909.

Smith, Henry Justin. Deadlines. Chicago: Covici-McGee, 1923.

————. Josslyn. Chicago: Covici-McGee, 1924.

Tarkington, Booth. The Gentleman from Indiana. New York: Scribner's, 1915.

Twain, Mark. Editorial Wild Oats. New York: Harper & Brothers, 1905; reprint ed., New York: Arno Press, 1970.

White, William Allen. In Our Town. New York: Macmillan, 1915.

Whitlock, Brand. The Happy Average. Indianapolis: Bobbs-Merrill, 1904.

Whitman, Stephen French. Predestined. Afterword by Alden Whitman. New York: Scribner's, 1910; reprint ed., Carbondale: Southern Illinois University Press, 1974.

Williams, Ben Ames. Splendor. New York: Dutton, 1927.

Williams, Jesse Lynch. The Day-Dreamer. New York: Scribner's, 1906.

————. The Stolen Story and Other Newspaper Stories. New York: Scribner's, 1899; reprint ed., Freeport, N.Y.: Books for Libraries Press, 1969.

Williams, Sidney. An Unconscious Crusader. Boston: Small, Maynard, 1920.

Williams, Wayland Wells. Goshen Street. New York: Frederick A. Stokes, 1920.

Wilson, Grove. Man of Strife. New York: Frank-Maurice, 1925.


## Contemporary Newspaper Fiction

Auchincloss, Louis. The House of the Prophet. Boston: Houghton Mifflin, 1980.

Caputo, Philip. DelCorso's Gallery. New York: Holt, Rinehart & Winston, 1983.

de Borchgrave, Arnaud, and Moss, Robert. Monimbó. New York: Simon & Schuster, 1983.

_____. The Spike. New York: Crown, 1980.

Diehl, William. Chameleon. New York: Random House, 1981.

Gordon, Barbara. Defects of the Heart. New York: Harper & Row, 1983.

Granger, Bill. Schism. New York: Crown, 1981.

Holland, Jack. The Prisoner's Wife. New York: Dodd, Mead, 1981.

Hoyt, Richard. 30 for a Harry. New York: M. Evans, 1981.

Just, Ward. The American Blues. New York: Viking Press, 1984.

Katzenbach, John. In the Heat of the Summer. New York: Ballantine, 1982.

Mitgang, Herbert. Kings in the Counting House. New York: Arbor House, 1983.

_____. The Montauk Fault. New York: Arbor House, 1981.

Parker, Robert B. A Savage Place. New York: Delacorte/ Seymour Lawrence, 1981.

Wallace, Irving. The Almighty. Garden City, N.Y.: Doubleday, 1982.

Secondary Sources

Allen, Frederick Lewis. Only Yesterday. New York: Harper & Brothers, 1931; paperback ed., New York: Harper & Row, 1964.

Anderson, Maxwell. Quoted in "Son Recalls Playwright Father," Grand Forks (N.D.) Herald, June 22, 1983, p. 1B.

Asbury, Henry. Gem of the Prairie: An Informal History of the Chicago Underworld. New York: Knopf, 1940.

Aydelotte, William O. "The Detective Story as a Historical Source." Yale Review, Sept. 1949–June 1950, pp. 76–95.

Bagdikian, Ben H. The Media Monopoly. Boston: Beacon Press, 1983.

Bannister, Robert C., Jr. Ray Stannard Baker. New Haven: Yale University Press, 1966.

Barris, Alex. Stop the Presses!: The Newspaperman in American Films. South Brunswick, N.J.: A. S. Barnes, 1976.

Beer, Thomas. The Mauve Decade. Garden City, N.Y.: Garden City Publishing, 1926.

_____. Stephen Crane. New York: Knopf, 1923.

Bent, Silas. Ballyhoo. New York: Boni & Liveright, 1927.

Berry, Thomas Elliott. The Newspaper in the American Novel, 1900–1969. Metuchen, N.J.: Scarecrow Press, 1970.

Bessie, Simon Michael. Jazz Journalism. New York: Dutton, 1938; reprint ed., New York: Russel & Russel, 1969.

Bleyer, Willard Grosvenor, ed. The Profession of Journalism. Boston: Atlantic Monthly Press, 1918.

Blumenthal, Albert. Small-Town Stuff. Chicago: University of Chicago Press, 1932.

Blythe, Samuel G. The Making of a Newspaper Man. Philadelphia: Henry Altemus, 1912; reprint ed., Westport, Conn.: Greenwood Press, 1970.

Born, Donna. "The Image of the Women Journalist in American Popular Fiction, 1890 to the Present." Paper presented to the Committee on the Status of Women of the Association for Education in Journalism, East Lansing, Mich., Aug. 1981.

_____. "The Woman Journalist of the 1920s and 1930s in Fiction and in Autobiography." Paper presented to the Qualitative Studies Division of the Association for Education in Journalism, Athens, Ohio, July 1982.

Boyer, Richard Owen. "The Trade of the Journalist." American Mercury, Jan. 1929, pp. 17-24.

Boynton, H. W. "The Literary Aspects of Journalism." Atlantic Monthly, June 1904, pp. 845-51.

Britt, George. Forty Years--Forty Millions: The Career of Frank A. Munsey. New York: Farrar & Rinehart, 1935.

Cawelti, John G. Adventure, Mystery, and Romance. Chicago: University of Chicago Press, 1976.

Chambers, Julius. News Hunting on Three Continents. New York: Mitchell Kennerley, 1921.

Churchill, Allen. Park Row. New York: Rinehart, 1958.

Cobb, Irvin S. Exit Laughing. Indianapolis: Bobbs-Merrill, 1941; reprint ed., Detroit: Gale Research, 1974.

Colby, F. M. "Attacking the Newspapers." Bookman, Vol. XV, Aug. 1902, pp. 534-36.

Commager, Henry Steele. The American Mind. New Haven: Yale University Press, 1950.

Crawford, Remsen. "Aces of the Press." North American Review, Jan. 1929, pp. 109-16.

"Danger of the Sensational Press." Craftsman, Nov. 1910, pp. 211-12.

Downey, Fairfax. Richard Harding Davis: His Day. New York: Scribner's, 1933.

Dreiser, Theodore. "Out of My Newspaper Days." Bookman, Vol. LIV, Sept. 1921-Feb. 1922, pp. 208-17, 427-33, 542-50.

Dunne, Finley Peter. Observations by Mr. Dooley. New York: Harper & Brothers, 1902.

Edel, Leon. The Stuff of Sleep and Dreams: Experiments in Literary Psychology. New York: Avon Books, 1982.

Ellis, Elmer. Mr. Dooley's America: A Life of Finley Peter Dunne. New York: Knopf, 1941.

Emery, Edwin, and Emery, Michael. The Press and America: An Interpretive History of the Mass Media, 5th ed. Englewood Cliffs, N.J.: Prentice-Hall, 1984.

Epstein, Edward J. Between Fact and Fiction: The Problem of Journalism. New York: Vintage Books, 1975.

Filler, Louis. The Muckrakers. University Park: Pennsylvania State University Press, 1976.

Fowler, Gene. Skyline. New York: Viking Press, 1961.

Fuller, Sam. "News That's Fit to Film." American Film, Vol. I, no. 1, Oct. 1975, pp. 20-24.

Gans, Herbert J. Popular Culture and High Culture. New York: Basic Books, 1974.

"The Gentlemanly Reporter." Century, Nov. 1909, pp. 149-50.

Gerbner, George. "Teacher Image and the Hidden Curriculum." American Scholar, Winter 1972-1973, pp. 66-92.

Griffith, Thomas. The Waist-High Culture. New York: Harper & Brothers, 1959.

Hansen, Harry. Midwest Portraits. New York: Harcourt, Brace, 1923.

Hapgood, Norman. The Changing Years. New York: Farrar & Rinehart, 1930.

Harger, Charles Moreau. "The Country Editor Today." The Profession of Journalism. Ed. by Willard Grosvenor Bleyer. Boston: Atlantic Monthly Press, 1918.

Hart, James D. The Popular Book. Berkeley: University of California Press, 1963.

Hart, James E. Floyd Dell. Twayne's United States Author Series. New York: Twayne, 1971.

Hecht, Ben. A Child of the Century. New York: Simon & Schuster, 1954.

_____. Gaily, Gaily. New York: New American Library, 1963.

"Henry James on Newspaper English." Current Literature, Vol. 39, Aug. 1905, pp. 155-56.

Hoggart, Richard. The Uses of Literacy. London: Chatto & Windus, 1957.

Holtzman, Natalie F. "The Image of Women Journalists in the American Novel, 1898-1957." Matrix, Summer 1977, pp. 24-25, 31.

Howells, William Dean. "Shocking News." Harper's Magazine, Oct. 1913, pp. 796-99.

Hughes, Helen MacGill. News and the Human Interest Story. Chicago: University of Chicago Press, 1940; reprint ed., New Brunswick, N.J.: Transaction Books, 1981.

Irwin, Will. The Making of a Reporter. New York: Putnam's, 1942.

Johnstone, John W. C., Slawski, Edward J., and Bowman, William W. The News People: A Sociological Portrait of American Journalists and Their Work. Urbana: University of Illinois Press, 1976.

Jordan, Elizabeth G. Three Rousing Cheers. New York: Appleton-Century, 1938.

Juergens, George. Joseph Pulitzer and the New York World. Princeton: Princeton University Press, 1966.

Kael, Pauline. "Raising Kane," The Citizen Kane Book. Boston: Little, Brown, 1971.

Kalish, Philip A., and Kalish, Beatrice J. "The Image of Nurses in Novels." American Journal of Nursing, Aug. 1982, pp. 1220-24.

Kando, Tom. "Popular Culture and Its Sociology: Two Controversies." Journal of Popular Culture, Vol. IX, Fall 1975, pp. 439-55.

Kaplan, Justin. Mr. Clemens and Mark Twain. New York: Simon & Schuster, 1966.

Kazin, Alfred. "Three Pioneer Realists." Saturday Review of Literature, July 8, 1939, pp. 3-4, 14-15.

Kelly, R. Gordon. "Literature and the Historian." American Quarterly, May 1974, pp. 141-59.

Kimball, Penn. "Journalism: Art, Craft or Profession?" Professions in America. Ed. by Kenneth S. Lynn and the editors of Daedalus. Boston: Beacon Press, 1967.

Knight, Grant C. The Critical Period in American Literature. Chapel Hill: University of North Carolina Press, 1951.

_____. The Strenuous Age in American Literature. Chapel Hill: University of North Carolina Press, 1954.

Kramer, Dale. Heywood Broun. New York: A. A. Wynn, 1949.

Kunitz, Stanley J., and Haycraft, Howard. Twentieth Century Authors. New York: H. W. Wilson, 1942.

Langford, Gerald. The Richard Harding Davis Years: A Biography of a Mother and Son. New York: Holt, Rinehart & Winston, 1961.

Larrabee, Eric. The Self-Conscious Society. New York: Doubleday, 1960.

Lawrence, D. H. Studies in Classic American Literature. New York: Viking Press, 1964.

Lindsay, Malvina. "Jackdaw in Peacock's Feathers." American Mercury, Feb. 1929, pp. 192-200.

Lord, Walter. The Good Years. New York: Harper & Brothers, 1960.

Lyon, Peter. Success Story: The Life and Times of S. S. McClure. New York: Scribner's, 1963.

Lyons, John O. The College Novel in America. Carbondale: Southern Illinois University Press, 1962.

McCutheon, John T. Drawn from Memory. Indianapolis: Bobbs-Merrill, 1950.

McKeen, William. "Heroes and Villains: A Study of Journalists in American Novels Published between 1915 and 1975." M.A. thesis, Indiana University, 1977.

McKenzie, Vernon, ed. Behind the Headlines. New York: Jonathan Cape & Harrison Smith, 1931.

McQuail, Denis. Towards a Sociology of Mass Communications. London: Collier-Macmillan, 1969.

Macy, John. "Journalism," Civilization in the United States: An Inquiry by Thirty Americans. Ed. by Harold E. Stearns. New York: Harcourt, Brace, 1922.

Mann, Arthur, ed. The Progressive Era, 2nd ed. Hinsdale, Ill.: Dryden Press, 1975.

Marzolf, Marion. Up from the Footnote. New York: Hastings House, 1977.

May, Henry F.  The End of American Innocence.  New York:
Knopf, 1959; reprint ed., Oxford:  Oxford University
Press, 1979.

Mencken, H. L.  A Choice of Days.  Selected and with an
introduction by Edward L. Galligan.  New York:  Vintage
Books, 1981.

_____.  "Journalism in America."  A Gang of Pecksniffs.
Ed. by Theo Lippman, Jr.  New Rochelle, N.Y.:  Arling-
ton House, 1975.

_____.  "The Leading American Novelist."  Smart Set,
Jan. 1911, pp. 163-64.

Miller, Max.  I Cover the Waterfront.  New York:  Dutton,
1932.

Moore, William T.  Dateline Chicago:  A Veteran Newsman
Recalls Its Heyday.  Foreword by Robert Cromie.  New
York:  Taplinger, 1973.

Mott, Frank Luther.  American Journalism, 3rd ed.  New
York:  Macmillan, 1962.

Munsterberg, Hugo.  "The Case of the Reporter."  Mc-
Clure's Magazine, Feb. 1911, pp. 435-39.

"Newspaper Responsibility for Lawlessness."  Nation, Aug.
20, 1903, p. 151.

Nord, David Paul.  "An Economic Perspective on Formula in
Popular Culture."  Journal of American Culture, Vol.
III, Spring 1980, pp. 17-31.

Nye, Russel.  The Unembarrassed Muse.  New York:  Dial
Press, 1970.

O'Connor, Richard.  The Scandalous Mr. Bennett.  New
York:  Doubleday, 1962.

Ogden, Rollo.  "Some Aspects of Journalism."  The Profession of Journalism.  Ed. by Willard G. Bleyer.  Boston:
Atlantic Monthly Press, 1918.

"Our Chamber of Horrors." Outlook, Sept. 30, 1911, pp.
    261-62.

"Our Seventeenth 'Special.'" Journalist, Vol. 28, Dec. 15,
    1900, p. 276.

Paine, Albert Bigelow. Mark Twain, Vol. 1. New York:
    Harper & Brothers, 1912.

Pancoast, Chalmers Lowell. Cub. New York: Devin-Adair,
    1928.

Paracelsus. "Confessions of a Provincial Editor." The Pro-
    fession of Journalism. Ed. by Willard G. Bleyer. Boston:
    Atlantic Monthly Press, 1918.

Park, Robert E. "The Natural History of the Newspaper,"
    The City. Ed. by Robert E. Park, Ernest W. Burgess,
    and Roderick D. McKenzie. Chicago: University of
    Chicago Press, 1925.

Pelley, W. D. "Human Nature As the Country Editor Knows
    It." American Magazine, Nov. 1919, pp. 60-61, 210-14.

Phillips, Melville, ed. The Making of a Newspaper. New
    York: Putnam's, 1893.

Pollack, Norman. The Populist Response to Industrial Amer-
    ica. New York: Norton, 1962.

Pulitzer, Joseph. "The College of Journalism," North
    American Review, May 1904, p. 642.

Ralph, Julian. The Making of a Journalist. New York:
    Harper & Brothers, 1903.

Ravitz, Abe C. David Graham Phillips. Twayne's United
    States Authors Series. New York: Twayne, 1966.

Reid, Whitelaw. "Journalism As a Career" and "Recent
    Changes in the Press," American and English Studies,
    Vol. 2. London: Smith, Elder, 1914.

Rosebault, Charles J. When Dana Was The Sun. New York:
    Robert M. McBride, 1931; reprint ed., Westport, Conn.:
    Greenwood Press, 1970.

Rosenberg, Bernard, and White, David Manning, eds. Mass Culture. Glencoe, Ill.: Free Press, 1960.

_____, eds. Mass Culture Revisited. New York: Van Nostrand Reinhold, 1971.

Ross, Ishbel. Ladies of the Press. New York: Harper & Brothers, 1936.

Ross, Malcolm H. Penny Dreadful. New York: Coward-McCann, 1929.

Rossell, Dean. "Hollywood and the Newsroom." American Film, Vol. I, no. 1, Oct. 1975, pp. 14-18.

Santayana, George. "Justification of Art," Little Essays. New York: Scribner's, 1920.

Schudson, Michael. Discovering the News. New York: Basic Books, 1978.

Seldes, G. H., and Seldes, G. V. "The Press and the Reporter." Forum, Nov. 1914, pp. 722-25.

Seldes, Gilbert. "The People and the Arts," The Great Audience. New York: Viking Press, 1951.

Shaw, David. "On Arrogance and Accountability in the Press." Address presented at the University of Hawaii, March 8, 1983.

Shirer, William L. 20th Century Journey. New York: Simon & Schuster, 1976.

Shuman, Edwin L. Practical Journalism. New York: Appleton, 1903.

Sinclair, Andrew. Jack: A Biography of Jack London. London: Weidenfeld & Nicolson, 1978.

Skaardal, Dorothy Burton. "Immigrant Literature as Historical Source Material: Problems and Methods." Paper presented to European Association for American Studies, Amsterdam, Netherlands, April 1980.

Sklar, Robert. Movie-Made America. New York: Random
    House, 1975.

Smith, H. Allen. The Life and Legend of Gene Fowler.
    New York: William Morrow, 1977.

Smythe, Ted Curtis. "The Reporter, 1880-1900: Working
    Conditions and Their Influence on the News." Journalism
    History, Vol. 7, no. 1, 1980, pp. 1-9.

Spatz, Jonas. Hollywood in Fiction. The Hague: Mouton,
    1969.

Steffens, Lincoln. The Autobiography of Lincoln Steffens,
    Vol. 1. New York: Harcourt, Brace & World, 1931.

Stone, Melville E. Fifty Years a Journalist. Garden City,
    N.Y.: Doubleday, Page, 1922.

Strunsky, Simeon. "Two Kinds of Reporters." Century,
    April 1913, pp. 955-57.

Sullivan, Mark. The Education of an American. New York:
    Doubleday, Doran, 1938.

Sutton, Albert A. Education for Journalism in the United
    States from Its Beginning to 1940. Evanston, Ill.:
    Northwestern University Press, 1945.

Tebbel, John. George Horace Lorimer and The Saturday
    Evening Post. Garden City, N.Y.: Doubleday, 1948.

_____. The Life and Good Times of William Randolph
    Hearst. New York: Dutton, 1952.

Walker, Stanley. City Editor. New York: Frederick A.
    Stokes, 1934.

Wecter, Dixon. The Hero in America. New York: Scrib-
    ner's, 1941.

White, William Allen. The Autobiography of William Allen
    White. New York: Macmillan, 1946.

Woodress, James. Booth Tarkington. Philadelphia: Lip-
    pincott, 1954.

Woodward, Bob. Quoted in "Movies and the Press Are an Enduring Romance," by Jane Gross. New York Times, June 2, 1985, sec. 2, p. 19.

"Working on Space." Journalist, Vol. 7, March 31, 1888, p. 8.

Ziff, Larzer. The American 1890s. New York: Viking Press, 1968.

Zynda, Thomas H. "The Hollywood Version: Movie Portrayals of the Press." Journalism History, Vol. 6, no. 1, Spring 1979, pp. 16–25, 32.

# INDEX